Advanced Clinical Skills for GU Nurses

Advanced Clinical Skills for GU Nurses

Edited by
MATTHEW GRUNDY-BOWERS
JONATHAN DAVIES

John Wiley & Sons, Ltd

Other Wiley Editorial Offices

John Wiley & Sons Inc., 111 River Street, Hoboken, NJ 07030, USA

Jossey-Bass, 989 Market Street, San Francisco, CA 94103-1741, USA

Wiley-VCH Verlag GmbH, Boschstr. 12, D-69469 Weinheim, Germany

John Wiley & Sons Australia Ltd, 42 McDougall Street, Milton, Queensland 4064, Australia

John Wiley & Sons (Asia) Pte Ltd, 2 Clementi Loop #02-01, Jin Xing Distripark, Singapore 129809

John Wiley & Sons Canada Ltd, 6045 Freemont Blvd, Mississauga, Ontario, L5R 4J3, Canada

Wiley also publishes its books in a variety of electronic formats. Some content that appears in
print may not be available in electronic books.

Library of Congress Cataloging-in-Publication Data

Advanced clinical skills for GU nurses / [edited by] Matthew Grundy-Bowers, Jonathan Davies.
     p. ; cm.
  Includes bibliographical references and index.
  ISBN-13: 978-0-470-01960-3 (pbk. : alk. paper)
  ISBN-10: 0-470-01960-3 (pbk. : alk. paper)
  1. Nurse practitioners.   2. Clinical competence.   I. Grundy-Bowers, Matthew.
 II. Davies, Jonathan, RN.
  [DNLM: 1. Nursing Care – methods.   2. Sexually Transmitted Diseases – nursing.
 3. Physical Examination – methods. WY 153 A244 2006]

RT82.8.A38   2006
610.73092 – dc22   2006011410

A catalogue record for this book is available from the British Library
ISBN-13: 978-0-470-01960-3
ISBN-10: 0-470-01960-3

Typeset by SNP Best-set Typesetter Ltd., Hong Kong
Printed and bound in Great Britain by TJ International Ltd, Padstow, Cornwall
This book is printed on acid-free paper responsibly manufactured from sustainable forestry in
which at least two trees are planted for each one used for paper production.

Contents

Dedication

In memory of Joyce, dad and grandad

Acknowledgements

Matthew would like to thank his family and his partner Joel for all their patience and support during the creation of this book. He would also like to thank Caroline for pushing him and for all her encouragement during the difficult stages. He would like to give a big 'thank you' to all the contributors, because without their input there would have been no book, and to give special thanks to Jonathan for coming on board at such short notice, and because the skills he has contributed have made the reach and scope of the completed book so much the greater.

Jonathan would like to thank Matthew for the invitation to contribute to this book and his partner Shaun for his continued support.

Contributors

Michelle Arnold, RN, BA (Hons), MSc
Consultant Nurse for Sexual Health at Waltham Forest PCT/Whipps Cross University Hospital
Previously Practice Educator (Sexual Health), St George's Hospital, Tooting, in which role she had a strong clinical practice and education/development focus, Michelle also develops and delivers pre- and post-registration education at Kingston University. She developed a competency-based training and assessment tool for nurses (2001), and recently added to this for the health-care support worker role. Michelle presented her competency work at the London Network of Nurses and Midwives (formerly London Standing Conference) Sexual Health group. This led to development of an integrated career and competency framework for sexual and reproductive health nursing (a collaborative project, published by the Royal College of Nursing in 2004). Michelle currently co-chairs the London Sexual Health Group.

Her clinical background (she started in Medicine/Rheumatology) sparked an interest in sexually transmitted infections and sexual health. Michelle has been nursing in sexual health since 1996. Her educational background includes an MSc in Sexually Transmitted Infections/HIV from University College London/London School of Hygiene and Tropical Medicine; a BA (Hons) in Social Sciences and Administration University of London, Goldsmiths' College; an ENB 276 in caring for persons with genito-urinary problems and related disorders; an ENB 934 in caring for persons with HIV/AIDS; Fertility and fertility control (a contraception qualification) and an ENB 998 in Teaching and assessing in clinical practice.

Jane Bickford, MSc, BSc (Hons), RGN, DLSHTM, PG Diploma Health Promotion
Nurse Practitioner, John Hunter Clinic, Chelsea and Westminster Hospital
After graduating with a science degree in 1983 Jane worked in an analytical chemistry lab before entering the nursing profession in 1985. Following nurse training she worked for four years as a medical nurse. In 1992 Jane left the UK and worked on an inpatient HIV unit in New York City. In 1995 she returned to the UK and studied for the Post Graduate Diploma in Health Promotion at Southbank University. In 1996 she started to work in sexual health and qualified as a contraception nurse in 2001. She was awarded an MSc in sexually transmitted infections and HIV by University College, London in 2004. Jane is the nursing representative on the Herpes Simplex Advisory Panel

within The British Association for Sexual Health and HIV. Jane's main interest within sexual health is the effect of stigma associated with sexually transmitted infections, and she has presented both nationally and internationally her research regarding stigma and genital herpes infection. She is currently a nurse practitioner at the John Hunter Clinic at the Chelsea and Westminster Hospital.

Jennifer Browne, RN
Nurse Practitioner – Praed Street Project, The Jefferiss Wing,
St Mary's NHS Trust
Jennifer trained at University College Hospital and The Middlesex Hospital in central London as a Registered General Nurse, qualifying in 1994. She worked initially in acute admissions and accident and emergency at University College Hospital.

Jennifer's first post in sexual health was at St Thomas' Hospital, London, where she gained a solid foundation in sexual health and completed the ENB 934, the HIV and AIDS course. She then worked as a staff nurse at Archway Sexual Health Clinic for three years where she started to find her niche in sexual health, working with CLASH (Central London Action Street Health) based in Soho, a project set up to work with male and female sex workers and street homeless. At Archway Sexual Health Clinic she achieved the ENB 8901, reproductive and family planning course and the ENB 276, sexual health course. Jennifer moved to Barnet Hospital where she held the position of Sister/Outreach Worker for SHOC (Sexual Health On Call) for two and a half years. There she enjoyed a varied role, providing outreach services to local flats and brothels, establishing satellite blood-borne virus clinics in the local drug dependency service and working within the main sexual health clinic. She worked closely with the sister project SHOC Haringey and learned from their good work of setting up a drop-in project for street sex workers. In the renowned Tottenham Beat she was asked to assist to establish a satellite clinical service with St Ann's Sexual Health Department based in Tottenham, North London where she has been lead nurse for five years. Jennifer is currently a Nurse Practitioner at the Jefferriss Wing, St Mary's Hospital, London, working for the Praed Street Project. The Praed Street Project is a three-tier approach for women working in the sex industry providing outreach, drop-in and clinical services. It is a well-established project which she is proud to be working for and which she has helped develop and expand. Jennifer commences study for an MSc in Sexual Health and HIV in September 2006.

Grainne Cooney, BSc (Hons), RGN, RM
Asymptomatic Screening Nurse
Grainne qualified as a registered nurse in 1993 in Barnet College of Nursing and Midwifery. After working in a paediatric ward in Barnet General Hospital for a year she moved to St Thomas' Hospital London. Here she completed the

'Special and Intensive Nursing Care of the Newborn' course at the Nightingale School, King's College London while working in the neonatal intensive care unit there. In 1996 Grainne began her midwifery training at Queen Charlotte's Hospital London and completed her BSc (Hons) in Midwifery at Thames Valley University. After working at Queen Charlotte's for several years Grainne took six months out to travel around South-East Asia.

On her return Grainne qualified in Family Planning Nursing at Middlesex University in 2000 and worked in Northwick Park Sexual Health Clinic for two years. During this time she completed her sexual health training at Thames Valley University. Travelling was still on the agenda, and in 2002 Grainne took a year out to travel and work as a midwife in Australia. In 2003 she commenced working in the John Hunter Clinic at the Chelsea and Westminster Hospital. She is currently working there as a Trainee Nurse Practitioner in Sexual and Reproductive Health, with a special interest in Family Planning.

Yaswant (Ravi) Dass, RN, BA (Hons), MSc
Nurse Practitioner in Genito-urinary Medicine, Bart's and the London NHS Trust
Ravi qualified as a nurse in 1997 and spent the first four years of his career in various jobs within medical and surgical nursing. He started GUM nursing in 2001 and has spent the past two and a half years working as a Nurse Practitioner, firstly at St Mary's Hospital London and currently at Bart's and The London NHS Trust. Within GUM nursing he also worked as a Clinical Facilitator / Charge Nurse where he was responsible for staff training and development.

Ravi has recently completed an MSc in Sexually Transmitted Infections and HIV at University College London, and is currently undertaking the nurse prescribing course. He has already completed several ENB courses, including Teaching and Assessing in Clinical Practice, and has been delivering lectures on Thames Valley University's sexual health courses. Ravi was central in the development of GUM services for HIV-positive patients at St Mary's Hospital London, and is currently developing nurse-led services within his current post.

Jonathan Davies, RN, Dip HE, MA
Senior Lecturer in Sexual Health, Thames Valley University
Jonathan Davies currently works as a Senior Lecturer at Thames Valley University, West London. Jonathan graduated from the same University in 1998 and has worked primarily in the field of sexual health for much of his nursing career. Since graduating Jonathan has worked in a variety of roles, including Staff Nurse, Charge Nurse, Nurse Practitioner and more recently Clinical Nurse Manager of The Jefferiss Wing at St Mary's Hospital, London.

Jonathan has continued his education since qualifying as a nurse; he gained a Master's Degree in Health Law from the University of Hertfordshire and is currently studying for a Post Graduate Diploma in Teaching and Learning. Jonathan believes strongly in the role that nurses play in the provision of sexual health care and believes that this book lends itself to the future development of nursing in the field of Genito-urinary Medicine.

Cindy Gilmour, RN, PG Dip
Nurse Practitioner, Chelsea and Westminster
Cindy qualified as a Registered General Nurse in 1987. Following qualification she worked as a staff nurse in acute medicine for two years and then from 1989 to 1996 worked as a staff nurse in Accident and Emergency. In 1996 Cindy moved into Sexual Health nursing, and in 1999 became a Nurse Practitioner at The West London Centre for Sexual Health. In 2000 she undertook the MSc in Nursing and Midwifery (Advanced Nurse Practitioner pathway) and obtained a Post Graduate Diploma in 2003. Cindy also took the role of Charge Nurse at the West London for a year in 2001. Since working in Sexual Health Cindy has been involved in several projects, including being the Lead Nurse for an Outreach Clinic for vaccinations and syphilis screening for men who sell sex, and also setting up a clinic for women who have sex with women. She takes an active role in staff development and facilitates teaching and assessing in advanced asymptomatic screening and sexual history-taking. At present Cindy is an assessor on the RCN Distance Learning Sexual Health course, and she also teaches on the STIF (Sexually Transmitted Infection Foundation) course.

Matthew Grundy-Bowers, RN, BSc (Hons)
Consultant Nurse in Sexual Health and HIV, St Mary's NHS Trust
Matthew qualified as a nurse in 1992 at the age of 20, being one of the youngest students to qualify from the Brent and Harrow School of Nursing and Midwifery. Initially, he worked as a staff nurse in Trauma Orthopaedics, before moving into Sexual Health in 1994. Since starting as an outpatient Staff Nurse in GUM and HIV in 1994 he has worked in various roles: Health Adviser, Nurse Practitioner, Senior Nurse for Sexual Health and HIV and Advanced Nurse Practitioner. He has broad experience in sexual health, HIV and family planning and also has experience working with patients with sexual dysfunction.

Matthew has undertaken various courses, including genito-urinary medicine (ENB 276), HIV/AIDS (ENB 934), Family Planning (ENB 901), Teaching and Assessing (ENB 998), and Research (ENB 870), as well as the BASHH course in STIs and HIV. He completed a BSc (Hons) Professional Studies – Nursing in 2002 from Thames Valley University and is an independent (extended and supplementary) nurse prescriber. He is currently writing up his dissertation for his MSc Nursing (Advanced Nurse Practitioner – Adult) at City University.

He also lectures at Thames Valley University, teaching on sexual health courses as well as teaching on the BASHH STIF course and for the Diploma in Family Planning.

He led the development of the advanced practice forum, which started out as a pan-London organisation and then became part of the GUNA. He is currently the co-chair of the London Network for Nurses and Midwives: Sexual Health Group. He has presented at various conferences, including the international conference for nurse practitioners and the RCN sexual health conference.

Jane Hooker, RN, BHSc
Senior Health Practitioner, The Jefferiss Wing, St Mary's NHS Trust

New Zealand-born Jane completed her Nursing Bachelor's degree in 1995 at Auckland Technical University. In 1999, after working in different acute medicine fields such as CCU and A & E at North Shore Hospital in Auckland, she left New Zealand to do what all good antipodeans do and see the world. Shortly after arriving in London she started working in the Jefferiss Wing at St Mary's Hospital and realised that she had found her ideal field of nursing. Over the last seven years she has worked as an agency nurse, Junior Sister and Nurse Practitioner, and for the last three years as the Senior Health Practitioner for the SHIP (Sexual Health Information and Protection) team. Jane is now happily settled in North-West London. She lives with her partner and two cats, and has a daughter due in August 2006.

Debby Price, MSc, BSc, PGCEA, RGN, RHV, RM
Subject Head, Public Health Primary Care and Thames Valley University

Debby trained as a nurse and midwife before studying for a degree in Social Science and Administration at the London School of Economics. She then qualified as a Health Visitor and worked in North-West London. During this time she became interested in adolescent sexual health, working in a unit for pregnant schoolgirls and as a family planning nurse. She moved into nurse education in 1989, teaching pre- and post-registration nurses. She has been at Thames Valley University since 1994, at first as the programme leader for the BSc Health Promotion and the family planning course. During this time she completed her Master's degree in Health Studies and completed a small research project on young people's perceptions of family planning clinics as part of the course. Since 2000 she has been the Subject Head for the Public Health and Primary Care subject group. Her subject team run programmes and short courses in primary care, public health and health promotion, sexual health and the care of older people, as well as teaching on the pre-registration nursing programme. Her own research interests remain with public health and policy and sexual health.

Colin Roberts, RN, RM, BNurs, PGC Sexual Health, Grad Dip Ed, Msc
Lead Nurse Specialist, Jefferiss Wing Centre for Sexual Health, St Mary's
Hospital, London
Colin Roberts is a Registered Nurse and Midwife, who has worked in Sexual
Health in Australia and the UK since 1990 gaining experience in both acute
and community HIV and sexual health. In 1997 he became one of the first
Nurse Practitioners in Genito-urinary Medicine at the Jefferiss Wing, St
Mary's Hospital London. From January 2000 he was the Clinical Nurse
Manager for Sexual Health based at the Queen Elizabeth Hospital NHS Trust
in Woolwich, South-East London. His clinical role involved weekly clinics at
HMP Belmarsh, The Pitstop Clinic for MSM, and a hospital-based men's clinic.
He assisted in developing courses for the BSc pathway in sexual health for the
University of Greenwich, whilst an honorary lecturer.

In 2003 he worked on the development of RCN Distance Learning Programme on Sexual Health, and remains an assessor for this programme.

He is passionate about the enhanced role of nursing within sexual health,
and was one of the founding members of the London Standing Conference
for Nurses, Midwives and Health Visitors – Sexual Health Group. He has been
part of the RCN Sexual Health Forum since 2003. He returned to the Jefferiss
Wing in July 2006.

Sonali Sonccha, Dip Clin Pharm Pract, MrPharmS
Lead Pharmacist HIV Services, North Middlesex University Hospital
NHS Trust
Sonali trained at Manchester University and Brighton and Sussex NHS Trust
and qualified as a pharmacist (MrPharmS) in 1998. She completed a post-
graduate diploma in pharmacy practice at the University of London in 2003.
Sonali has worked as an HIV specialist for 6 years and currently works at the
North Middlesex University Hospital NHS Trust, where she is the Lead
Pharmacist HIV Services. Her role includes running patient adherence clinics,
management of the drugs budget, audit work and guidelines development, as
well as inpatient care. She also sits on the HIV Pharmacy Association steer-
ing committee, where she represents HIV pharmacy at a national level, organ-
ising training days and developing CPD initiatives with sponsors.

Previously, Sonali worked at Bart's and the London NHS Trust, initially as
a rotational pharmacist and then as a GUM and HIV specialist. Her role
included providing advice on the appropriate use of medicines, aiding in the
set-up of new GUM services (a sexual assault centre, for example), clinical
audit, financial management of GUM drugs budgets and the writing of GUM
drugs guidelines. She was also involved in developing PGDs for use in GUM
clinics and in training nursing staff in their use. Sonali has earlier taught on
the City University postgraduate nursing course in HIV/GUM and has trained
both junior and undergraduate pharmacists and physicians in GUM and HIV
medication issues.

Foreword

Poor sexual health is now a major public health issue in the UK, with all four countries having a sexual health strategy, strategic framework or action plan in place. The Government in England wishes to improve sexual health services, with a focus on improving access.

All over the country nurses are working in new and innovative ways in sexual and reproductive health. Many are working in advanced and specialist clinical roles as independent practitioners and more creative posts are being developed in the National Health Service to maximise optimum use of nurses' skills. Several Nurse Consultant posts have now been developed in the speciality of Genito Urinary Medicine (GUM).

With this important public health agenda in mind, this book provides a valuable resource for nurses working towards, and at, advanced level in GUM, but the content is also transferable and relevant to nurses working in non-acute settings.

This book also provides a skill base for more junior nurses in GUM to aspire to. Using a competency-based approach, many GUM nurses could develop their practice to an advanced level, using nurse prescribing and/or patient group directions to complement the level of service they provide.

I welcome the publication of this book, as I firmly believe, that historically there has never been a better time for nurses to develop their roles in GUM and sexual health, to drive forward improvements and to lead service delivery in this challenging, changing and dynamic area of health in the twenty-first century.

Anita Weston
Nurse Consultant in Genito Urinary Medicine
Guy's and St Thomas' NHS Foundation Trust
London
July 2006

1 Defining Advanced Practice

MATTHEW GRUNDY-BOWERS

INTRODUCTION

This is a very exciting time to be a nurse and in sexual healthcare. Deteriorating sexual health in the United Kingdom (UK), with increases in bacterial and viral sexually transmitted infections, including HIV, are putting a huge strain on sexual health services (PHLS, 2002). This has caused two things to happen. Firstly, in an attempt to improve patient throughput, a number of services are reviewing and challenging practices that have been around for years. For example, some clinics have stopped undertaking microscopy on asymptomatic women, while others have stopped urethral gonorrhoea cultures in asymptomatic patients. Perhaps this challenge to existing practice might not have happened without the increased burden on clinics. Secondly, nurses and other healthcare professionals are examining and redefining their roles in order to meet the increasing demands on clinical services. This has caused role delineation to become blurred as doctors, nurses and health advisers adapt their practice to meet these demands whilst constrained by both financial and environmental pressures.

Early in 2005, the Nursing and Midwifery Council (NMC) (NMC, 2005) conducted a consultation about the registration of a second level of practice beyond that of initial registration. It acknowledges that some nurses are working at a different (advanced) level and that registration of this would offer the public great protection. There was also a consultation by the Medicines and Healthcare products Regulatory Authority (MHRA) (MHRA, 2005) in 2005 looking at the extended nurse prescribers' formulary. This was because there were a number of problems with the limited formulary. There were anomalies, which caused confusion, and the formulary was not responsive to changing healthcare practice. To keep abreast of these changes meant that the formulary had to be reviewed regularly, which was expensive and time-consuming. This deterred a number of nurses and pharmacists from undertaking the course, as it didn't meet the needs of a large number of prescribers. Following the consultation an announcement was made in November 2005 by the Department of Health that extended nurse prescribers would be able to prescribe any licensed medicines for any medical condition with the exception of controlled

Advanced Clinical Skills for GU Nurses. Edited by Matthew Grundy-Bowers and Jonathan Davies
© 2007 John Wiley & Sons Ltd

drugs from spring 2006 onwards (DH, 2005). This is obviously going to have a huge impact on the way advanced practice nurses in sexual health work.

Finally, both sexual health and nursing in general have been in the spotlight. This began with *The NHS Plan* (DH, 2000), followed by *The National Strategy for Sexual Health and HIV* (DH, 2001) and its implementation plan (DH, 2002). There was also a position statement from the Sexual Health Working Group of the London Standing Conference for Nurses, Midwives and Health Visitors (LSC, 2002), the Sexual Health Competencies, competency framework for nurses in sexual health (RCN, 2004) and *Effective Commissioning for Sexual Health Services* (DH, 2003), the House of Commons Health Select Committee report on sexual health services (Health Select Committee 2003), and the public white paper *Choosing Health: Making Healthy Choices Easier* (DH, 2004). Finally, in 2005 came the Medfash *Recommended Standards for Sexual Health Services* (2005) and the BASHH *standards for sexual health services* consultation document (BASHH, 2005), all of which have placed nursing and sexual health very much on the national agenda.

Therefore, in order to define advanced practice this chapter will:

1. Briefly explore the main drivers that explain why healthcare delivery is changing;
2. Explore contemporary nursing roles;
3. Examine the difference between specialist and advanced practice;
4. Document the history of advanced practice;
5. Define advanced practice and the educational preparation thereof; and
6. Discuss the future.

THE CURRENT DRIVERS FOR CHANGE

As has been mentioned previously, since 1997 the NHS has been subject to extensive reform and modernisation. Government policy has directed attention towards not only nursing but also sexual health as well. The most important themes that run through all these developments are the vital contribution of nursing and the evolution of innovative nursing roles. This chapter is not going to discuss each of these drivers in any great detail, as nurses in sexual health are well versed in most of the documents. They can also be found on the Internet if people want to explore them further. However, it would be prudent to discuss the main documents that have affected advanced nursing practice in sexual health in a little more detail.

MAKING A DIFFERENCE AND THE NHS PLAN

Making a Difference (DH, 1999) and *The NHS Plan* (DH, 2000) set out the groundwork for advanced nursing practice. *Making a Difference* mentioned pregnancies, as well as a doubling in GUM clinic attendances in England over the preceding ten years. The strategy was produced as part of a nationwide programme of investment and reform, to modernise services around the needs of patients and service users. It aimed to tackle inequalities in service provision and ensure that the NHS works to prevent ill health. It was drawn up in line with the principles of *The NHS Plan* (DH, 2000) (see above), and by involving service users and experts from across the country allowed clients to have a real say. Unlike *The Health of The Nation* (1993), which had to be achieved within existing budgets, the strategy was accompanied by extra investment of £47.5 million over a two-year period.

The strategy hoped to reach its aims (see Box Two) by delivering evidence-based effective local HIV/STI programmes so that people could make informed decisions about preventing STIs, including HIV, and by setting a target to reduce the number of newly acquired HIV infections. It also hoped to increase the offer and uptake of HIV testing to reduce the number of undiagnosed people with HIV in the UK, as well as increasing the offer and uptake of hepatitis B vaccine, both of which policies came with specific targets.

It highlights collaborative working between providers so that they deliver a more comprehensive sexual health service to patients and sees a broader role for those working in primary-care settings. The strategy also sets out a new way of working in which there will be three levels of service provision (see Table 1). The strategy acknowledges that for good practice level one service should be universally provided in General Practice, but that level two will also be provided by some general practitioners that have a 'special interest' in sexual health as well as in family planning clinics. Departments of sexual and reproductive health and HIV will provide the specialist level three services.

This comes at a time when GPs are over-stretched, and with practice nurses and primary-care nurse practitioners already providing contraceptive care (LSC, 2002) it is natural to assume that their roles will be expanded to incorporate these recommendations. It has been suggested that nurses working in primary care already provide advice and health promotion around sexual health issues (LSC, 2002). Alternatively, GP practices may employ sexual health nurse practitioners to undertake clinical sessions for them.

Box Two

Aims of the national strategy for sexual health and HIV (DH, 2001)
• reduce the transmission of HIV and STIs • reduce the prevalence of undiagnosed HIV and STIs • reduce unintended pregnancy rates • improve health and social care for people living with HIV • reduce the stigma associated with HIV and STIs

Table 1 Levels of practice (DH, 2001)

Level One	• Sexual history and risk assessment • STI testing for women • Assessment and referral of men with STI symptoms • HIV testing and counselling • Contraceptive information and services, including cytology screening, pregnancy testing and referral • Hepatitis B immunisation
Level Two	• All of Level One plus: • Intrauterine device (IUCD) insertion, vasectomy, contraceptive implant insertion • Testing and treating sexually transmitted infections, including partner notification and invasive STI testing for men
Level Three	• All of Levels One and Two plus: • Outreach for sexually transmitted infection prevention • Outreach of contraception services • Specialised infections management, including co-ordination of partner notification • Highly specialised contraception • Specialised HIV treatment and care

Plans exist to increase access by providing a choice of easily available services and exploring the benefits of more integrated sexual health services, including piloting of one-stop clinics. If these mirror the format of NHS walk-in centres, they may well be nurse-led.

The sexual health strategy states that:

'The growing role of nurses within the NHS generally is likely to be mirrored in sexual health practice' (DH, 2001, p. 46).

The strategy placed great emphasis on the importance of open access to genito-urinary services and, over time, improving access for urgent appointments. This is at a time when sexual health services especially are at breaking point. Open-access services are changing to appointments-only to better manage their ever-increasing workload, which has the knock-on effect of limiting access. Walk-in services commonly now shut the doors early because of the large volumes of service users, and four-hour waits are common. For departments to work shorter waiting times for urgent appointments and increasing access they will have to make better use of nurses' skills and abilities, and the strategy acknowledges this:

'Nurse   have an expanded role ... as specialists and consultants' (DH, 2001, p. 26).

According to the position statement from the London Standing Conference for Nurses, Midwives and Health Visitors (Sexual Health Group) (LSC, 2002) an estimated 65 per cent of London departments of GUM already have nurses providing autonomous, first-line STI management.

This raises implications for the training, development and education of the workforce, which it plans to address across the whole range of sexual health and HIV services:

'The development of nurse referral and prescribing, and of nurse specialists and nurse consultants, raises issues for their training and ongoing education.' (DH, 2001, p. 46).

Currently, there are no specific advanced practice Genito-urinary nurse practitioner courses: therefore how will nurses acquire the skills and knowledge to achieve the objectives of the strategy? Also, since the demise of the Boards of the four countries there is no single recognised validating body for nursing courses. This leaves us with many inconsistencies; for example, each university may offer a variety of sexual health courses with varying content and assessment methods.

The NMC's consultation document suggests that this type of practice is clearly advanced: therefore will all practice nurses who deliver level one services need to undertake a Master's degree in order to implement the strategy? Will Genito-urinary nurses working at levels two and three need to be advanced nurse practitioners? Or is this really specialist practice? As we can see, there are many questions still to be answered.

CONTEMPORARY NURSING ROLES

Next it would be important to explore contemporary nursing roles in the UK. Currently in the UK 'advanced practice nurses' have many titles and roles. For evidence of this one just needs to flick through recent copies of the job sections of nursing magazines. Nurses undertaking the same role may have different titles, and nurses with the same title are often practising at different levels or even performing different jobs (Ibbotson, 1999). The titles 'nurse practitioner', 'nurse clinician', and 'clinical nurse specialist', to name but a few, are often used interchangeably (Manley, 1997) and this use of multiple titles is cause for concern (Wright, 1997). Confusions as to levels of practice and their required educational preparations bewilder both nurses and managers alike (Wright, 1997; McCreaddie, 2001). For example some nurse practitioner posts are banded at 5–6, and require little more than initial undergraduate education, while others are banded at 8B, and require a Master's-prepared nurse. Patients and other healthcare professionals are perplexed by this myriad of roles and titles (Ormond-Walshe & Newham, 2001), as they often don't know what to expect from the healthcare practitioner sitting in front of them.

These challenges are mirrored in the nursing literature, where assumptions are made regarding titles and their implied levels of practice. For example because they share the same basic role components (Ormond-Walshe & Newham, 2001) 'Clinical Nurse Specialist' and 'Nurse Practitioner' are often referred to in terms of both specialist and advanced practice. Even when looking at research about nurse practitioner roles, very little reference was made to 'defining' what was meant by 'advanced practice'. This makes discussing roles and levels of practice difficult, owing to inconsistencies among the titles and grades (Cattini & Knowles, 1999). Therefore it would be important to establish what is meant by these terms and discuss the difference between them.

THE CLINICAL NURSE SPECIALIST

It is suggested by Hunt (1999) in the UK nurses have 'specialised' since the Nightingale era. But the Clinical Nurse Specialist role as it is today began to appear in the United States in the 1930s. It didn't reach the UK until the 1980s, and has continued to evolve across a wide range of specialties (Bousfield, 1997). Although role development has been *ad hoc* (Gibson & Bamford, 2001), it was expected that one should have considerable experience in the field and a post-registration qualification. In the USA Clinical Nurse Specialists are educated to Master's degree level, and it is considered that they are 'advanced practice nurses'. Gibson and Bamford (2001) suggested that there is a lack of evidence in the UK to support Master's education for nurse specialists, while Bousfield proposed (1997) that the literature suggests that, for role recognition to occur, practitioners would need to be educated to an advanced level. A brief appraisal of the literature yields a broad consensus of opinion on the key components of the Clinical Nurse Specialist role, identifying the four main themes as follows: clinical, consultative, educational and research roles.

However, some of the other components that were identified from the literature were those of Role Model (Wright, 1997), Leader (Bousfield, 1997), Patient Advocate (Wright, 1997; Bousfield, 1997), Change Agent (Ormond-Walshe & Newham, 2001; Wright, 1997), Developer of Procedures and Protocols (McCreaddie, 2001) or Administrator (McCreaddie, 2001; Gibson & Bamford, 2001). These other very different key components could be attributed, as was mentioned earlier, to the fact that specific aspects of the role would depend on the practice setting and client group (Kleinpell, 1998). Sidani & Irvine (1999) did, however, determine that prescribing pharmacological ᵗˢ was beyond the Clinical Nurse Specialist's scope of practice.

NURSE PRACTITIONERS

HISTORICALLY

Nurse practitioners are now common, and practice in a number of specialties (Le-Mon, 2000) from accident and emergency (Shea & Selfridge-Thomas, 1997) to dementia care (Rolfe & Phillips, 1995). In a postal survey of 17 closed-response questions by Miles *et al.* (2002) to identify and describe nurse-led clinics in genito-urinary medicine services across England, of the 209 Departments across England 190 responded (a 91% response rate). The author showed that some nurses had taken on 'nurse practitioner' roles including eliciting the sexual history, performing the examination, making a diagnosis, and supplying selected treatments.

Le-Mon (2000) proposed that development of the nurse practitioner role had been hampered by its lack of structure and that role definition was important for it to be accepted in the healthcare community. Sidani and Irvine (1999), who suggest that there is variability in role conceptualisation and that role responsibilities are unclear, supported this view. The title of 'nurse practitioner' had not been protected (Le-Mon, 2000), and the former UKCC didn't see the nurse practitioner role as an advanced practice role because of its medicalisation (Casey, 1996). The UKCC (1993) believed it to be ambiguous, as all nurses 'practise': hence all nurses are nurse practitioners.

DEFINING WHAT A NURSE PRACTITIONER IS

Often criticised by non-nurse practitioners as being 'mini doctors' and not nurses (Woods, 1998), the nurse practitioners' key strength comes from the utilisation and augmentation of both sets of skills in clinical practice. They assess both the bio-medical and psycho-social (nursing) facets involved in caring for their client group, rather than adopting a cure-only perspective (Mundinger, 1995). In a sense, then, they combine the best of both worlds (Ventura, 1998) and are described as 'hybrids' that 'blend' (Mick & Ackerman, 2000), and 'integrate' both expanded nursing functions and medicine into their clinical practice (Sidani & Irvine, 1999). This is better described by Le-Mon (2000), who suggests that doctors assess health, using a natural science perspective in relation to standardised norms where health is the absence of disease, and nurses utilise a holistic approach in which only individuals can describe their own health. It is because of this approach that the nurse practitioner's emphasis is on preventive health care and health promotion (Ventura, 1998), although, they must retain a nursing core with its focus on 'care', rather than adopting the medical model with its focus on 'cure' (Wright, 1997).

The Royal College of Nursing (2005) stated that nurse practitioners make professionally autonomous decisions, for which they have sole responsibility, and receive patients/clients with undifferentiated and undiagnosed problems. An assessment of their healthcare needs is made on the basis of highly developed nursing knowledge and skills. This includes special skills not usually exercised by nurses, such as physical examination. They screen patients for disease risk factors and early signs of illness. In conjunction with the patient they develop a nursing care plan for health with an emphasis on preventive measures, and provide counselling and health education. Nurse practitioners also have the authority to admit and discharge from their own caseloads and to refer to other healthcare providers as appropriate.

The *American Academy of Nurse Practitioners Scope of Practice* position statement states that nurse practitioners are advanced practice nurses who provide primary health care and specialised health services to individuals, families, groups and communities (AANP, 1993). Mundinger (1995) suggests that in primary care doctors and nurse practitioners share common bases of knowledge, and that while doctors obviously have a greater depth of knowledge around disease detection, nurses also bring different additional skills. These include a holistic health assessment, which incorporates environmental and family factors, health promotion/education, disease prevention, counselling and the knowledge needed to craft a care regimen using community and family resources.

CONSULTANT NURSES

The consultant nurse posts were first set out in the *Making a Difference* document (DH, 1999). More detailed guidance was issued in Health Service Circular 1999/217. Nurse consultants are important new leadership positions. Reaching the position allows nurses to remain in practice doing what they came into nursing to do. The consultant nurse role was developed as an alternative career path for experienced and senior nurses who otherwise might have entered management or have gone into higher education or have left the profession to retain contact with patients (NHS Executive, 1998). Consultant posts represent the pinnacle of the clinical career structure. Appointees are experienced practitioners with advanced education and qualifications in the specialty to which they are appointed. The role has four key functions: expert practice; professional leadership and consultancy; education, training and development; and practice and service development and research and evaluation (see Box Three).

Elcock (1996) suggests that consultant nurses are advanced practitioners, sharing the same roles, skills and characteristics. The role is concerned with adjusting boundaries; it is a catalyst for change and is a pioneer for strategic development, which is based on research. Therefore the consultant nurse and advanced practitioner share similar sub-roles and skills (Manley, 1997).

Box Three

The four key functions of a consultant nurse

The expert practice function

- As expert clinicians nurse consultants will spend 50% of their time in direct clinical practice.

The professional leadership and consultancy function

- To support and inspire colleagues
- Improve standards and quality
- Have a crucial role in clinical governance
- Influence other disciplines and the wider organisation and exert influence across organisations to help deliver better services.

The education, training and development function

- To identify and respond to learning needs at individual, team and organisational levels
- Develop advanced knowledge and skills in experienced colleagues
- Develop links and productive partnerships with Universities
- Play a key role in leadership and professional development

The practice and service development, research and evaluation function

- Develop practice local and national
- Promote evidenced-based practice
- Be at the forefront of practice and innovation
- Generate, monitor and evaluate practice protocol
- Help plan and shape services
- Undertake research to support practice

SPECIALIST PRACTICE AND ADVANCED PRACTICE

So what is specialist and advanced practice and is there a difference between them? Up until recently in the UK, PREP (UKCC, 1995) identified two levels of practice beyond registration which are specialist and higher (UKCC, 1995; Rolfe & Phillips, 1995). This has been further superseded by the NMC (2005) which is now looking to register 'advanced practice' nurses.

SPECIALIST PRACTICE

The term 'specialist' is used to denote anyone who is more 'experienced' or more specialised than oneself (Hunt, 1999). Most of the literature when discussing 'specialist practice' does so in relation to the clinical nurse specialist role. Other countries, such as the USA, see the terms 'specialist', 'expert' and 'advanced' practice as synonymous with each other (Sutton & Smith, 1995), so it is impossible to draw on their experiences. In the absence of specific literature on specialist practice as a level of practice, guidance is taken from the former UKCC (1998). Cattini and Knowles (1999) identified a framework of core competencies for specialist practice, which are: be a clinical expert in direct clinical practice; deliver research-based practice; act as a clinical resource for patients and staff; and be able to manage the workload and act as an effective communicator. In clinical practice, care management, practice development and leadership specialist practitioners exercise higher levels of judgement, discretion and decision-making (UKCC, 1998).

THE EDUCATIONAL PREPARATION FOR SPECIALIST PRACTICE

The UKCC (1998) defined very specific requirements for recording specialist practitioners. They are first level registration and completion of a programme of educational preparation over at least one academic year that consists of 50 per cent clinical work and 50 per cent practice that is at degree level. This is supported by Humphris (1994) (cited by Cattini & Knowles, 1999) who suggests that the education of specialist practitioners should be at degree level. The entry criteria are normally two years experience and a diploma in nursing (Norman, 2000). The UKCC also set out various educational standards for 'specialist practice' for different clinical areas, such as community learning, disabilities nursing and health visiting. New clinical posts that adapt what were previously medical tasks are primarily 'specialist practice' roles if they fulfil the criteria for specialist practice (Elcock, 1996; Manley 1997), and the UKCC agreed that nurse practitioners or clinical nurse specialists could use the title if they met the standards (Norman, 2000).

Examining the standard for specialist community nursing education and practice – general practice nursing (points 15–16) from the UKCC 1998 standard clearly demonstrates that managing episodes of care in the way they would be managed by nurses in sexual health fulfils the criteria for 'specialist' practice:

16.2 assess, diagnose and treat specific disease in accordance with agreed medical/nursing protocols

16.3 provide direct access to specialist nursing care for undifferentiated patients within the practice population

˙ˑˑndertake diagnostic, health screening, health surveillance and therapeutic techn˦ˑˑˑ ˑnlied to individuals and groups within the practice population.

(UKCC, 1998)

ADVANCED PRACTICE

Clearly, these points could also easily apply to advanced practice. However, advanced practice is substantially different from other forms of nursing practice such as expert or specialist practice (Sutton & Smith, 1995). It is a pinnacle of nursing that is more than a collection of extended roles (Le-Mon, 2000) and breaking it down into parts would fail to capture the essence of the role (Elcock, 1996). Advanced practice transcends roles: it is a way of thinking and approaching new challenges with vision and acting as a catalyst for change (Davies & Hughes, 2002). In meeting organisational demands, advanced practitioners are 'eclectic', which is probably why there is role ambiguity (Woods, 1999). Clinical expertise in a related sphere of practice is essential (Manley, 1997), as advanced practice is grounded in the nurse–client relationship (Sutton & Smith, 1995). Advanced practice is independent and should be performed without reference to doctors or protocols (Sidani & Irvine, 1999). Advanced practice nurses also demonstrate a level of analytical thought that shapes their perception of practice, and articulate and define nursing practice by constant reference to the client (Sutton & Smith, 1995).

Worldwide, the delivery of health care is changing, and to meet that challenge nurses are adapting their practice and developing advanced practice roles (Mundinger, 1995; Lorensen *et al.* 1998; Offredy 2000). Although it is useful to explore how advanced practice is developing in other countries such as the USA, which has had these roles for years, drawing from those experiences, it is important to note that advanced practice is defined by the reasons for its development. As there is no clear definition (Davies & Hughes, 2002), describing advanced practice becomes a complex issue. There has been much discussion here in the UK and overseas about the nature and standard of advanced practice (Elcock, 1996; Woods, 1999).

USA

In the USA advanced practice is synonymous with clinical nurse specialists and nurse practitioners (Davies & Hughes, 2002). It is suggested that it is a level of practice that includes but is not exclusive to these roles (Wright, 1997). The development of the 'strong' model of advanced practice, by a group of advanced nurse practitioners in America in 1994, gave clear guidelines as to what the characteristics of advanced practice were. It incorporates comprehensive care, education, and research and publication, and also professional leadership (Mick & Ackerman, 2000).

Australia

In Australia there appears to be debate as to whether blind adoption of the 'American model' is the correct way to go (Offredy, 2000). Interestingly the

Australians are looking to the UK model of specialist and higher-level practice. The Australians identified as far back as 1992 that nursing resource should be better utilised, but practitioners were constrained by legal barriers and took steps to change this.

Canada

The Canadian perspective, however, is somewhat different (de Leon-Demare *et al.,* 1999). Canada followed the USA in its development of advanced practice roles. Owing to chronic shortages the Canadian government had to look to alternatives to physician-directed care. The advanced practice nurse was seen as a cost-effective alternative healthcare provider and was developed to improve access to preventive primary care, especially for the underserved, remote rural areas. This, however, led to advanced practice nurses being stigmatised as being replacement physicians. When the shortage of doctors was reversed there was a backlash against advanced practice.

Scandinavia

The Nordic experience of advanced practice is very different from the UK, Canadian and US perspectives. This is because they have had no shortage of doctors; therefore nurse practitioner roles that are based on the acquisition of 'medical roles' have not been developed. Advanced practice is seen as a 'higher level' of generalist nursing practice, and strives to improve quality while reducing costs (Lorensen *et al.,* 1998). This is similar to the description of 'higher-level' practice as laid down by the former UKCC (1999).

Higher level practice

At this point it would be useful to discuss higher-level practice (UKCC, 1999), despite the fact that it has been replaced, as it has some useful points which shouldn't be lost. Higher-level practice was similar to the Nordic experience of advanced practice, because it is about nursing research to assist nurses in a productive, practical, applicable way (Lorensen *et al.,* 1998). Practitioners working at a higher level understand the social, economic and political implications of health care. They use complex reasoning, critical thinking, and reflective skills, and are able to analyse and synthesise information by generating new solutions. They contribute to the wider development of nursing through publication, and are leaders for change. Effective communicators, they network, and cross organisational and professional boundaries to ensure collaborative working and to develop practice standards and protocols. They are clinical experts who work in the absence of procedure and protocols. They ~ssess risk and promote clinical effectiveness. So with higher-level practice it was ~ a matter of acquiring medical skills such as health assessment, and they may have been nurses who would not fit into the 'advanced nurse practitioner' as defined by the NMC but may contribute at a 'higher level' than an initial registration-level nurse. The advanced practice nurse and consultant nurse are characterised by similar sub-roles (Manley, 1997).

The educational preparation for advanced practice

Historically, much of the debate about educational preparation for advanced practice was really about whether nurse practitioners were advanced practice nurses. When you take nurse practitioners out of the equation, in the UK there is little doubt that advanced practitioners should be educated to Master's level (Elcock 1996; Wright, 1997; Manley, 1997), a view which is now supported by the NMC (2005). There is a consensus that the key components of the role would be expert practitioner, educator, researcher and consultant (Elcock, 1996). This is because advanced practitioners are involved in the breaking down of existing professional barriers and redefining practice parameters and contributing to health policy. This level of critical thinking and decision-making, and analytical skills, can only be achieved through a Master's level educational preparation (Davies & Hughes, 2002). This is similar to the educational preparation in the USA (Mick & Ackerman, 2000), and in the Nordic countries. In the Nordic countries advanced practice education focuses on nursing research, addressing nursing science issues such as confusion, anxiety, incontinence, sleep and pain, and all of these are addressed from multiple perspectives. There they also believe that preparation for advanced practice should be at Master's level to enable the nurse to synthesise nursing research; their programmes run over three years and prepare practitioners to lead and manage health care, to teach and develop research-based clinical expertise (Lorensen *et al.*, 1998).

So what is advanced practice?

This question raises a number of issues. Having looked at the literature there still appears to be confusion about what 'advanced practice' is. Advanced practice is not about the acquisition of skills that doctors would normally have. It is important to differentiate advanced *clinical* skills from advanced nursing practice, as they are not one and the same and they cannot be used interchangeably. That is not to say that a number of nurse practitioners are not also advanced practice nurses; but by mixing the two we are in danger of losing the essence of nursing by placing value on non-nursing activities.

Historically, nurse practitioners have been advanced practice nurses. This is because the posts have been about changing traditional boundaries and challenging the status quo. Therefore the people who took these posts would have to have been advanced practice nurses. However, now, further down the line, these roles are established and commonplace, so that they don't necessarily require the same skills from the post-holder. Again, this is not to say that all post-holders are not as capable as before; just that the requirements to work successfully in these posts are now different. Because of this it is important to say that the registration of advanced nurse practitioners is an important and significant step, which is generally well supported. However, advanced practice is more than that: as Le-Mon (2000) suggested, it is a pinnacle of nursing that is more than merely a collection of extended roles.

It is also important to remember that most advanced clinical roles globally have evolved from a shortage of doctors. In some countries like Canada (de Leon-Demare *et al.,* 1999), when that shortage is reversed there is a huge backlash against these roles. Therefore it is important to co-develop advanced practice roles that don't place overmuch value on the acquisition of medical skills such as physical assessment, and to utilise existing models such as the Nordic experience (Lorensen *et al.,* 1998), which consists purely of 'higher-level' nursing skills and knowledge based on nursing research that improves nursing care for patients, and not nursing theory, which is often perceived by nurses as being abstract and unrelated to practice.

THE FUTURE

In the UK, as in the USA, there seems to be a recent shift towards bringing Clinical Nurse Specialists and Nurse Practitioners together under the same title of 'Advanced Nurse Practitioner' (ANP). This potentially welcome shift fits in with the plans in the United Kingdom to register ANPs (NMC, 2005), and this will do a number of things. Firstly, it will provide patients and other healthcare professionals with a clear message of what to expect from this level of nurse. It will also provide nurses with a clear understanding of what educational preparation and what clinical competency is needed. Finally, it will reduce the number of titles used in practice. For example, within the sexual health clinical setting the 'HIV clinical nurse specialist' might become 'advanced nurse practitioner (HIV)' and 'genito-urinary nurse practitioners' may become 'advanced nurse practitioners' (GUM). These practitioners will share a common educational preparation and more importantly a common registration.

REGISTRATION OF ADVANCED NURSE PRACTITIONERS

At the time of writing this chapter the NMC had not finalised the finer details about how this registration will happen. Therefore the following is speculation ... at the NMC will suggest. There will be a transitional phase until 2010, which w... existing practitioners the opportunity to gain the components to register. Pe... the way that it will work is that during the transitional phase nurses will have to demonstrate two things to the NMC to become registered: (1) they will have to demonstrate Master's-level education in a health-related subject; and (2) they will have to demonstrate competency in the National Organisation of Nurse Practitioner Faculties (NONPF) competency framework through a portfolio of learning. This might mean that some practitioners, who already hold an MSc, might have to pick up other modules, such as a physical assessment module or nurse prescribing.

THE NATIONAL ORGANISATION OF NURSE PRACTITIONER FACULTIES (NONPF) COMPETENCY FRAMEWORK

As well as demonstrating Master's-level education, nurses wanting to be registered as an 'advanced nurse practitioner' with the NMC will have to demonstrate that they have met the competencies adapted by the RCN (2005) (although these may be subjected to minor changes before use by the NMC). These domains and competencies are based on the work of the NONPF in America, who developed the original competencies in 1995, and have been revised a number of times since then. The RCN based their domains on the 2001 version. The competencies are a framework for nurse practitioners to base their practice on. Aspiring nurse practitioners will need to demonstrate competence in these via a portfolio of learning.

THE FUTURE REGISTRATION OF ANPS

Ultimately, there will be a specifically designed advanced nurse practitioner Master's degree course, with a curriculum that is set by the NMC in the same way as is done with pre-registration courses, and which all future advanced nurse practitioners will have to attain prior to registration. The course content would most likely follow that of the existing nurse practitioner programmes from North America. Like other nursing programmes, the course would be 50 per cent clinical and 50 per cent theoretical, and it might include the following modules; physical assessment, research, advanced clinical practice, health promotion/education, and leadership and would be based on the acquisition of competency in the RCN domains of practice (see Box Four). It could also be postulated that independent extended and supplementary nurse prescribing would also be linked to this qualification; however, this might not be an 'essential' requirement, as some advanced practice nurses may not in their roles need to prescribe. The courses would be generic, leading to advanced nurse practitioner (adult), advanced nurse practitioner (child), etc. There would either be specialist 'optional' modules in the Master's programme, such as HIV or Sexual Health, or further certification on completion of the ANP course in a specialist field would be required. For example, one might be an

Box Four

The RCN domains of practice (RCN, 2005)

1. Management of patient health/illness status
2. The nurse–patient relationship
3. The teaching and coaching function
4. Professional role
5. Managing and negotiating healthcare delivery systems
6. Monitoring and ensuring the quality of healthcare practice
7. Cultural competence

---

advanced nurse practitioner (adult), PG Cert. Sexual Health. This approach may well allay the fears of some of our medical colleagues who voice concerns about Nurse Practitioners' clinical ability. It could also mean that permission to apply these skills in clinical practice would not be dictated by the preference of the lead medical consultant of a service or the senior nurse.

CONCLUSION

We have seen that there are a number of drivers, predominantly in the form of government reforms, that are guiding this explosion of advanced nursing practice. Nurses are a flexible and adaptable workforce within the health service, and it is this flexibility that has facilitated this role development. Because of this change and nursing initiative there has been a phenomenal development of nursing roles, which has led to there being a number of titles used by advanced practice nurses, which has confused both other healthcare professionals and patients alike. This was fuelled by a lack of direction from the former UKCC, who avoided regulating this practice.

Finally, this chapter aimed to define what 'advanced nursing practice' is. This has proved to be a difficult task. There is a perception that it consists in the development of medical skills such as health assessment. It is easy to understand why: these are indeed 'advanced clinical skills'. However, advanced nursing practice is more than a collection of medical skills. It is about challenging the status quo of what nurses have traditionally been expected to do, and developing clinical practice in which the patients' needs are central. It could be suggested that a ward sister or other senior nurses could practise at this 'advanced level', even though they may not possess advanced clinical skills such as health assessment or nurse prescribing. This is important to remember when discussing advanced nursing practice, or otherwise the value of nursing could be lost at the expense of learning these exciting new clinical skills. In summary it would be fair to say that currently in the UK there are three levels of practice, not two, and these are initial, specialist and advanced.

With all this in mind this book is concerned with helping nurses acquire and develop these exciting new advanced clinical skills in genito-urinary medicine, with the aim that many of them will go on to become advanced nurse practitioners.

REFERENCES

AANP (American Academy of Nurse Practitioners) (1993) *Nurse Practitioners as an Advanced Practice Nurse Position Statement*. AANP, Austin TX
BASHH (British Association for Sexual Health and HIV) (2005) *Consultation for the Standards for Sexual Health Services*. BASHH, London
Bousfield C (1997) A phenomenological investigation into the role of the clinical nurse specialist. *Journal of Advanced Nursing* Vol. 25(2) 245–56 (February)
Casey N (1996) Editorial. *Nursing Standard* Vol. 10(49) 1
Cattini P, Knowles V (1999) Core competencies for Clinical Nurse Specialists: a usable framework. *Journal of Clinical Nursing* Vol. 8(5) 505–11 (September)
Davies B, Hughes A (2002) Clarification of Advanced Nursing Practice: Characteristics and Competencies. *Clinical Nurse Specialist* Vol. 16(3) 147–52 (May)
de Leon-Demare K, Chalmers K, Askin D (1999) Advanced practice nursing in Canada: has the time really come? *Nursing Standard* Vol. 14(7) 49–54 (November 3)
DH (Department of Health) (1993) *The Health of the Nation*. DH, London
DH (Department of Health) (1999) *Making a Difference: Strengthening the Nursing Midwifery and Health Visiting Contribution to Health and Healthcare*. DH, London
DH (Department of Health) (2000) *The NHS Plan*. DH, London
DH (Department of Health) (2001) *Better Prevention, Better Services Better Sexual Health – The National Strategy for Sexual Health and HIV*. DH, London
DH (Department of Health) (2002) *The National Strategy for Sexual Health and HIV Implementation Action Plan*. DH, London
DH (Department of Health) (2003) *Effective Commissioning for Sexual Health Services*. DH, London
DH (Department of Health) (2004) *Choosing Health: Making Healthy Choices Easier*. DH, London
DH (Department of Health) (2005) *Nurse and Pharmacist Prescribing Powers Extended*. Press Release Reference Number 2005/0395 DH, London
Elcock K (1996) Consultant Nurse: an appropriate title for the advanced nurse practitioner? *British Journal of Nursing* Vol. 5(22) 1376–81
Gibson F, Bamford O (2001) Focus group interviews to examine the role and development of the clinical nurse specialist. *Journal of Nursing Management* Vol. 9(6) 331–42 (November)
Health Select Committee (2003) Sexual Health Third Report of Session 2002–2003. The Stationary Office, London
Humphris D (1994) *The Clinical Nurse Specialist: Issues in Practice* Macmillan, London

Hunt J (1999) A specialist nurse: an identified professional role or a personal agenda? *Journal of Advanced Nursing* Vol. 30(3) 704–12 (September)

Ibbotson K (1999) The role of the clinical nurse specialist: a study. *Nursing Standard* Vol. 14(9) 35–8 (November)

Kleinpell, R (1998) Reports of role descriptions of acute care nurse practitioners. *AACN Clinical Issues* Vol. 9(2) 290–5 (May)

Le-Mon, B (2000) The role of the Nurse practitioner. *Nursing Standard* Vol. 14(21) 49–51 (February)

Lorensen M, Jones DE, Hamilton GA (1998) Advanced practice nursing in the Nordic countries. *Journal of Clinical Nursing*. Vol. 7(3) 257–64 (May)

LSC (London Standing Conference for Nurses, Midwives and Health Visitors) (2002) Challenges and opportunities for sexual health nursing in London: a position statement from the sexual health working group. NHS London Regional Office, London

Manley K (1997) A conceptual framework for advanced practice. An action research project operationalising an advanced nurse practitioner/consultant nurse role. *Journal of Clinical Nursing* 6 179–90

McCreaddie M (2001) The role of the clinical nurse specialist. *Nursing Standard* Vol. 16(10) 33–8 (November)

Medfash (Medical Foundation for Sexual Health and HIV) (2005) *Recommended Standards for Sexual Health Services*. Medfash, London

MHRA (Medicines and Healthcare products Regulatory Agency) (2005) Consultation on Options for the Future of Independent Prescribing by Extended Formulary Nurse Prescribers (mlx 320). http://www.dh.gov.uk/assetRoot/04/10/40/58/04104058.pdf (accessed 12/06/2005)

Mick D, Ackerman M (2000) Advanced practice nursing role delineation in acute and critical care: application of the Strong Model of Advanced Practice. *Heart & Lung: The Journal of Critical Care* Vol. 29(3) 210–21 (May)

Miles K, Penny N, Mercey D, Power R (2002) A postal survey to identify and describe nurse-led clinics in Genito-urinary medicine services across England. *Sexually Transmitted Infections* Vol. 78(2) 98–100 (April)

Mundinger M (1995) Advanced Practice Nursing is the Answer . . . What Is the Question? *N&HC: Perspectives on Community* Vol. 16(5) 254–9 (Sept/Oct)

NHS Executive Health Service Circular (1998) Nurse Consultants HSC 1998/161 (22nd September)

NMC (Nursing and Midwifery Council) (2005) *Consultation on a Framework for the Standard for Post-Registration Nursing*. NMC, London

NMC (Nursing and Midwifery Council) (2005) *NMC News* (July)

Norman S (2000) Making sense of higher-level practice. *Nursing Standard* Vol. 14(35) 49–51 (May)

Offredy M (2000) Advanced nursing practice: the case of nurse practitioners in three Australian states. *Journal of Advanced Nursing* Vol. 31(2) 274–81 (February)

⌐Walshe S, Newham R (2001) Comparing and contrasting the clinical nurse spec⌐   ⌐the advanced nurse practitioner roles. *Journal of Nursing Management* Vol. 9(4) 2⌐⌐

PHLS (Public Heal⌐⌐   ⌐ory Service). Communicable Disease Surveillance Centre, HIV/STI Division ⌐⌐   ⌐*⌐l Health in Britain: Recent Changes in High*

Risk Sexual Behaviours and the Epidemiology of Sexually Transmitted Infections Including HIV. PHLS. Colindate, London http://www.hpa.org.uk/infections/topics_az/hiv_and_sti/publications/sexual_health.pdf (accessed 12/06/2006)

RCN (Royal College of Nursing) (2004) Sexual Health Competencies: *An Integrated Career and Competency Framework for Sexual and Reproductive Health Nursing.* RCN, London

RCN (Royal College of Nursing) (2005) *Nurse Practitioners – An RCN Guide to the Nurse Practitioner Role, Competencies and Programme Approval.* RCN, London

Rolfe G, Phillips L (1995) Action research project to develop and evaluate the role of an advanced nurse practitioner in dementia. *Journal of Clinical Nursing* Vol. 4(5) 289–93 (September)

Shea S, Selifridge-Thomas J (1997) The ED nurse practitioner: pearls and pitfalls of role transition and development. *Journal of Emergency Nursing* Vol. 23(3) 235–7 (June)

Sidani S, Irvine D (1999) A conceptual framework for evaluating the nurse practitioner role in acute care settings. *Journal of Advanced Nursing* Vol. 30(1) 58–66 (July)

Sutton F, Smith C (1995) Advanced nursing practice: new ideas and new perspectives. *Journal of Advanced Nursing* Vol. 21(6) 1037–43 (June)

UKCC (United Kingdom Central Council for Nurses, Midwives and Health Visitors) (1993) *Final Draft Report on the Future of Professional Education and Practice.* UKCC, London

UKCC (United Kingdom Central Council for Nurses, Midwives and Health Visitors) (1995) *Standards for Post-Registration Education and Practice.* UKCC, London

UKCC (United Kingdom Central Council for Nurses, Midwives and Health Visitors) (1998) *Standards for Specialist Education and Practice.* UKCC, London

UKCC (United Kingdom Central Council for Nurses, Midwives and Health Visitors) (1999) *A Higher Level of Practice – Pilot Standard.* UKCC, London

Ventura M (1998) NPs vs. MDs. *Registered Nurse* Vol. 61(2) 27–9 (February)

Woods L (1998) Implementing advanced practice: identifying the factors that facilitate and inhibit the process. *Journal of Clinical Nursing* Vol. 7(3) 265–73 (May)

Woods L (1999) The contingent nature of advanced nursing practice. *Journal of Advanced Nursing* Vol. 30(1) 121–8 (July)

Wright K (1997) Advanced Practice Nursing: Merging the Clinical Nurse Specialist and Nurse Practitioner Roles. *Gastroenterology Nursing* Vol. 20(2) 57–60 (March/April)

2 Taking a Sexual History

COLIN ROBERTS

WHAT IS A HISTORY?

In the context of a health consultation a history is the recollection of events that have gone before and precede the current encounter. For our purposes it is a narrative, the person's story that we are recording for the purposes of aiding in a health assessment.

WHY DO WE NEED A SEXUAL HISTORY?

The rationale for obtaining a sexual history is straightforward. As a healthcare worker you need to be able to undertake an assessment of the risk of the person's acquiring a sexual infection or an unintended pregnancy, or continuing to live with a sexual problem that affects their life (Jones & Barton, 2004). The history will guide the staff as to the most appropriate investigations, the treatment required and the correct follow-up for the person and their partner(s) (Barone & Becker, 1999). A key aspect of every history-taking process is the ability to inform and teach the person, promoting his or her own sexual health and independence (Evans, 2004). If the process is handled effectively and the condition is curable we may never see the person again.

WHAT DO YOU NEED?

The practitioner requires good skills in communication, and most importantly the ability to listen to what is being said. Don't just listen to **what** is being said, but to **how** it is being said. You will learn a lot from the tone, speed and volume of the conversation. Fear, embarrassment or anger may be demonstrated in the way that the person is interacting with you. You must be aware of why you are asking the questions and what is the significance of the responses that are obtained (Clutterbuck, 2004). This is explained later in the chapter.

The other key skills that are required are a comprehensive knowledge of the common sexually acquired infections/conditions. This will include the signs,

Advanced Clinical Skills for GU Nurses. Edited by Matthew Grundy-Bowers and Jonathan Davies
© 2007 John Wiley & Sons Ltd

symptoms and transmission routes. You should be able to link the symptoms being described to a potential diagnosis, and you must be aware of the range of tests that you have available to you, with the turnaround time for results (Jones & Barton, 2004).

You will also need a room or space where you can talk privately and openly; this can be an issue in some hospital areas or clinics. You must be able to provide somewhere where you will not be overheard or interrupted if your history-taking is to be accurate (Potter & Flory, 2004).

SETTING THE SCENE

The initial twenty to forty seconds will usually set the tone for the consultation, so it is important that you minimise the risk of any misunderstandings (Law & McCoriston, 1996).

Do not assume, just because you are seeing a person in your clinical setting, that the person knows where they are (Clutterbuck, 2004). From the author's experience some people have waited for up to two hours in a clinic that they thought was for the dentist. Those for whom English is not their first language or who have no previous experience can misinterpret the acronym 'GUM'.

Depending on where you are working, the system for booking in people may differ; however, the key steps that you should include are: introduce yourself, confirm the person's identity, explain briefly what you are about to do and why, and stress the confidentiality that covers the process (Clutterbuck, 2004).

CULTURAL COMPETENCE

It is very important that as a nurse you are aware of the profound cultural issues with which we may have to deal. It is very important that you do not cause offence or insult the person sitting with you as a result of a lack of thought on your part (Green, 1999; Meacher, 1999; Law & McCoriston, 1996).

Be aware of the major cultures that are represented in your local area. Is it appropriate that you interview this person if there is a gender difference? In Australia, it would be totally inappropriate for a male healthcare worker to ask an Australian Aboriginal woman about 'women's business', that is, sexual health, menstrual history or contraception (Bell, 1998). In the Muslim culture men may not be willing to have an examination performed by a woman. If in any doubt check it out with your colleagues or indeed carefully ask the person *'Is it appropriate that I ask you questions about your sexual health? Would you prefer that I get my male colleague to see you today?'* You can usually sense the person's discomfort immediately and/or if the body language indicates a defensive posture.

Be aware of the local users of your service, this is especially important if you work with young people or marginalized groups, such as people who are regular drug users. This will influence the terminology that you should be aware of, such as '*works*' for needle and syringes. This will facilitate clearer communication between you and your clients (Clutterbuck, 2004; Green, 1999).

You cannot know all the street language or sub-cultural language used, so ask your client if there is any doubt. As well as broadening your own vocabulary, this aids in *rapport*-building with the person – you are actively engaging them to help you understand. One of the major barriers that you can erect between you and the client is using judgemental language, which at best irritates them, and at worst alienates them, so that your interview may fail (Meacher, 1999; Clutterbuck, 2004; Green, 1999).

The list below is a sample of the terms of which you must be aware:

- Drug abuser vs. drug/substance user
- Prostitute vs. sex worker, working girl/boy
- Affairs vs. sexual contacts
- Promiscuous vs. more than one sexual partner.

Law & McCoriston (1996)

There are several styles of taking a sexual history and you will develop your own style with experience and practice. It is very important that you use language that you are comfortable with and understand. Familiarise yourself with the terminology used in sexual health settings and where possible either sit in with an experienced colleague or at least watch one of the health education videos available (Clutterbuck, 2004; Green, 1999). There have been a number of helpful videos produced, which will help you understand how to obtain a history in a variety of settings (Law & McCoriston, 1996).

One of the most damaging things that you can do as a healthcare worker is to make assumptions about the person with whom you are working. This can lead to the person's not being provided with the most appropriate screening, nor indeed the correct treatment. There is nothing wrong with trusting your instincts; however, always be mindful of the biases that may impact on your practice (Law & McCoriston, 1996). Examples of these are the ideas that all homosexually active men engage in anal sex or all people who inject drugs are chaotic people who steal to fund their habit.

The order in which you conduct your history-taking is a personal one. What is important is that you have a structure to follow. A good example of a framework is 'The Enhanced Calgary–Cambridge Guide to the Medical Interview' (Kurtz *et al.*, 2003).

The two major styles commonly seen in sexual health can be described as follows. The non-confrontational 'gentle' approach is to ask the generic components of any health history first. The consultation progresses from the introduction to the general medical history and the social history, and leaves the sexual history until the end. This technique allows you to build up *rapport* with the person and get a general view of their life story prior to asking the 'intimate' questions, which may be embarrassing.

Conversely, some clinicians believe that if you are working in a sexual health context the person has come to ask/tell you about a sexual issue, and therefore not to ask about it first may appear to the person as lack of interest. In this format, after the introduction the clinician moves directly into the collection of the sexual history, followed by the other components (Clutterbuck, 2004; Green, 1999).

Remember that you must use the style which suits you and the setting in which you work, as there is no absolute way. You may alter your approach according to the age, cultural background and other social information available; this is particularly important if the person is coming to see you after a sexual assault (Law & McCoriston, 1996). You must ensure the dignity and privacy of the person at all times and, if a question appears to have upset them, clarify it and explain why you need to know the answer.

Clinicians are often worried about how to find out the gender of a person's sexual partner without causing offence to the person. Some clinicians will use non-gender-specific terms when requesting information about a client's sexual contacts or relationships. You must be careful and ensure that you do establish the gender of the sexual partners, bearing in mind that some people will have both male and female partners. Some clinicians will use *'What is your partner's first name?'* This is immediately problematic, especially if the response is gender-neutral, for example, 'Chris', as this could be a Christine or a Christopher. Cultural variance can also lead to ambiguity: therefore you must politely validate the gender. If you have set the scene with your initial introduction, asking these questions should cause little offence (see the sample history proforma below) (Clutterbuck, 2004; Green, 1999; Temple-Smith *et al.*, 1998).

QUESTIONING STYLES

There are two major types of questions used in sexual history taking, the 'open' and the 'closed' variety. It is usual to use a mixture of both in the context of a sexual history. Try to avoid the overuse of one style, as using nothing but closed questions can feel like an interrogation. Conversely, using nothing but open questions can lead to a very long consultation if the interviewee is prone to being talkative (Kurtz *et al.*, 1998; Tomlinson, 1998). Examples of open questions might include:

'Could you tell me why you have come to see us today?'
'What do you think has caused the problem?'

These will usually lead to an explanation of the issue in the person's own words, which can lead to clues for further investigation.

Examples of closed questions include:

'Do you have pain when you pass urine?'
'Did you use a condom?'

The responses are often a simple 'yes' or 'no', which allows you to gather significant amounts of information in a short time.

There is debate about the use of colloquial language, mirroring the language of the client. The interview is an opportunity for education as well as problem-solving, and the author believes that as a professional you need to assist the interviewee to tell you their story. *'When you say screwing her, do you mean your penis in her vagina?'* The use of this style may assist the person in future visits with your service, as they may pick up the terms you have used to describe how they have sex with their partner (Clutterbuck, 2004; Green, 1999; Law & McCoriston, 1996).

Try to avoid the use of the medically correct terms for sexual practice, as they are so rarely used outside textbooks or theoretical lectures. An example of this would be *'his penis in your mouth'* rather than *'fellatio'* or *'your tongue in her vagina'* rather than *'cunnilingus'*.

If you have not had the opportunity to learn about sexual practices before, familiarise yourself now with all the things people can do in enjoying a full sex life, as well as the language that is used to describe each of them. Here are a few examples:

- Skin to skin – body rubbing, frottage
- Oral contact – fellatio, cunnilingus
- Oro-anal contact – rimming
- Vaginal intercourse – penis in vagina
- Digital sex – fingers in vagina/anus
- Anal intercourse – penis in anus
- Use of pleasure devices/'sex toys' – dildos, vibrators
- Others, for example 'fisting' – fingers leading to hands in the rectum or vagina.

When you are working with people you need to be aware that it is what they have done that puts them at risk of acquiring an infection, not the particular social group to which they belong. Check for behaviours that may have put them at risk. Do not assume that your client is automatically at risk if they belong to what the public may identify as a 'risk group'. When seeing men and women who present themselves as gay, remember to check for possible further sexual contact with the opposite sex (Clutterbuck, 2004; Law & McCoriston, 1996; Verhoeven *et al.*, 2003).

WHY HAS THE PERSON COME FOR A CHECK-UP?

People may come forward for a health screening for a number of reasons. These may include the fact that they have never had a screen and feel it is time that they did; that they have a partner with whom they wish to stop using condoms, so that they have both agreed to undergo screening; that they now have symptoms that they don't usually have, and are therefore worried; that they have had a recent exposure and want peace of mind; or they may be engaging in screening prior to fertility treatment or prior to taking out a mortgage or an insurance policy; or their partner may have been at risk, and they have come in for screening as a contact (Presswell & Barton, 2000).

Your initial questions should identify why the person has come for a check-up. Be aware that there may be a subtext to their visit: careful listening will help you identify if there are other concerns (Law & McCoriston, 1996; Presswell & Barton, 2000). These may include sexual dysfunction: therefore follow up throwaway lines or ambiguity – '*So does this cause impotence?*' Your response may be '*Is impotence or problems with having sex worrying you?*'

The following is a breakdown of typical questions that are asked (and a brief rationale for the use of them) during a sexual history consultation at Genitourinary Medicine or Sexual Health Clinics in the United Kingdom. It should be remembered that the depth of questioning that follows may not be appropriate for or indeed suitable in a generalist setting owing to constraints of time or the nature of the patient group (Clutterbuck, 2004; Green, 1999; Law & McCoriston, 1996).

You can adapt the questions to fit in with your own situation.

THE WELCOME

Greet the person by their name. Check that you have the right person and the correct date of birth. Introduce yourself and what your role is; clarify that the consultation is confidential and that you will be taking brief notes. Explain that some of the questions that you will ask in working out what the problem might be are by their nature necessarily quite personal. You will only be asking questions that will help you work out what the problem might be. The questions you ask are asked of all people who attend the clinic/surgery for a sexual health check.

THE INTERVIEW

Start off with some open-ended questions that will allow the person to tell you in their own words what has brought them to make the appointment.

'What has brought you to see me today (use their first name, e.g. 'Peter', 'Natalie')?'

Or

'How may I help you today (use their first name, e.g. 'Peter', 'Natalie')?'

Or

'Let's start by you telling me about what's brought you to see me today (use their first name, e.g. 'Peter', 'Natalie').'

Paraphrase and record what they tell you. Using their first name indicates that you are talking personally with them.

'Has this ever happened before?' (Is it therefore a first occurrence or is this a chronic problem for which they have not sought help before? *Are there any systemic symptoms?* (For example, fever, myalgia/arthralgia?) *If it has happened before, is it the same as before?* (Briefly describe: is it worse or the same or indeed getting better?)

'When do you notice the symptoms?' (For example, is there pain on passing urine?)

'Who did you see for this last time?' (Briefly describe: it may be the GP or a Family Planning Clinic.)

'Did they give you any treatment?' (If yes – did it ever go away? Briefly describe.)

'Have you tried any self-treatment?' (If so, what have they tried and what was the outcome? This will give you a good idea of why the person has come and give you some clues as to the potential infection and your subsequent management. You may now either go straight into the sexual history or start with the more generalist health questions.)

RECENT SEXUAL HISTORY

'When did you last have sexual contact with someone?' (Describe briefly, for example the week as x/52, the month as x/12: this helps you ascertain the incubation periods for infections as well as the window period for HIV and hepatitis.)

'Was this person male or female?' This will guide your questioning and assist you in the risk assessment. Please remember that if the client is female and having sex with another woman this doesn't necessarily mean that they are not at risk: that other woman may have had male relationships in the past and may have acquired chlamydia, genital warts or HIV. The use of shared sex toys may also be a risk factor.

'Is this your regular partner, or someone you know, or was it a casual contact?' If it is a regular partner they may already know if the partner has

signs or symptoms of an infection. If it is a casual contact this can help with your health promotion later and aid in partner notification. Describe using the sexual health abbreviations if you are comfortable with their use, e.g. Regular Male Partner (RMP), Regular Female Partner (RFP), Known Male Partner (KMP), Known Female Partner (KFP), Casual Male Partner (CMP), and Casual Female Partner (CFP).

'*What type of sex did you have?*' (You may need to prompt or clarify – 'vaginal sex, that is your penis in her vagina', 'oral sex, that is his penis in your mouth', 'anal sex, that is his penis in your anus', 'mutual masturbation', etc. This helps you establish the relative risks.

'*Which country do they come from?*' – This gives you important clues in establishing the relative risks of potential infections/conditions that you might need to think about, e.g. tropical infections, or syphilis.

'*Did you use condoms?*' (If yes, any splits, breaks or other problems with condoms? If no: 'Do you usually use condoms' – record the result, and be aware that some people may not have used condoms initially but put them on later. You need to make them aware that they are still at risk for acquiring a sexual infection.

'*Is your partner using another form of contraception?*' (Describe – is pregnancy an issue that you need to be aware of?)

'*When did you last have sexual contact with someone different?*' (Repeat as above.)

Be aware that some clients will have more than one regular partner. This can be a cultural issue: for example some people will have a person who has borne their child that is their baby mother, but she may not be the only regular sexual partner. This is important in partner notification. Condoms may only be used with people other than the baby mother. If contacts are all casual or your intuition suggests multiple partners, clarify, for instance 'How many partners in the last three months (3/12)?'

'*Could you give me an idea of how many different partners you have had, say in the last 3 months?*' (Record the answer in a form that helps in your risk assessment, e.g. '7 CMP oral sex only', '2 KFP all protected', or '0 condoms', 'with & without condoms', 'x3 split', etc.)

'*Have you ever been told that you have had a sexual infection in the past?*' – Record yes/no. If yes when, and ask which one(s): this will give you assistance in a clinical diagnosis, such as a recurrent lesion that could be herpes.

'*Where did you get treated?*' – Identify the hospital or the country. This is important for assessing the type of treatment given.

'*Did you go back for follow up?*' Record response.

'*Was/were your partner(s) treated at the same time?*' – Record yes/no, and describe if the treatment was the same for both. This gives you a lot of information that may guide your differential diagnosis, help with treatment options, and assist in partner notification. It may be a failed treatment or a re-infection from a non-treated/incompletely treated partner.

GENERAL HEALTH ASSESSMENT

'How would you describe your health in the past?' – Paraphrase what they tell you. Ask for any specific chronic problems, such as diabetes, asthma, epilepsy, or skin problems that can affect their sexual health either directly or as a result of medication.

'Have you had any surgery?' – You define for yourself if it is major or minor and whether a blood transfusion may have been given. Record how long ago, especially if before 1985 in the UK.

IF FEMALE

'When was your last menstrual period?' – This gives you information about possible pregnancy, other hormonal problems or pituitary problems.

'Do you have any problems with your periods – pain, heavy loss, etc.?' – Record the response.

'Do you use any form of contraception?' – Describe and clarify if you haven't obtained this during the sexual history section. Describe any problems that they may disclose.

'How many pregnancies have you had?' – This gives information on sexual activity, usage of contraception or ability to negotiate safer sex.

'How many live births?' – Although the question is self-explanatory, it may disclose multiple miscarriages, termination of pregnancies, neonatal deaths, and previous genital infection, which in some cases can lead to miscarriage.

'Are all your children alive and well?' This may disclose medical issues such as HIV or congenital problems. *'What ages are they now?'* This may help with your HIV risk assessment if testing was offered in the antenatal check-up. (NB: This is not an essential question.)

'When was your last cervical smear?' – If she has not had one within the last three years, give a brief reason for regular smears and explain briefly that the best way to obtain one is with her GP. If your screening is not being undertaken in the GP surgery, you may not wish to do the smear.

'Have you been asked to re-attend sooner than the usual three years follow-up?' – Describe briefly if there is shorter recall.

FAMILY MEDICAL HISTORY

'In your family – that is, your parents, brothers and sisters – are there any health problems that seem to run through the family?' You may prompt with suggestion such as diabetes, hypertension, and skin problems. This gives you information about predisposition, especially with diabetes and skin problems, and helps with differential diagnosis and may be a contributing factor in the reason for the visit, as for example with impotence or recurrent vaginal candidiasis.

GENERAL MEDICAL HISTORY

'Are you allergic to any tablets, foods or medicines?' Record what they tell you and remember this for what treatment they may receive.

'Are you currently taking any tablets or medicines, including any tablets not prescribed by your doctor?' Record any regular medicines: this is important, as some health food products, for example St John's Wort, will potentiate other medicines. If you get the names of medications used in specific conditions you may need to amend your previous entries – for example, lithium usually indicates a psychiatric condition – clarify with the client.

RISK ASSESSMENT

'Do you have any tattoos?' – If yes, you want to know if they were professionally done in this country or if they were done outside of a regulated facility, as there is an increased risk of blood-borne infections if they were done in a non-regulated facility.

'Do you have any body piercing?' If yes, you want to know if it was professionally done in this country or if it was done outside of a regulated facility, as there is an increased risk of blood-borne infections if it was done in a non-regulated facility.

'Have you ever injected drugs for any reason?' If yes, you want to know if they have ever shared, and when was the last time that they used/shared. Which drugs did/do they use? Be aware that you may not get this information if they do not trust you and/or the use that may be made of this information in the future.

Regular use of drugs may increase the risk for HIV and hepatitis and the ability to practise/negotiate safer sex. You may ask about willingness to be referred for support.

'Do you use any recreational drugs?' Which drugs did/do they use? Be aware that you may not get this information if they do not trust you and or the use that may be made of this information in the future. Regular use of drugs may increase the risk for HIV and hepatitis and the ability to practise/negotiate safer sex: for example, snorting coke can cause nose bleeding and lead to blood-to-blood transmission of hepatitis (Fieldhouse, 2005).

'Have you ever been given blood in a transfusion?' Record when and where, if it hasn't been given in the response to any of the major health problems above. This gives you information about the potential for blood-borne infections, as all donations have been tested since 1985. It will also help you establish the three-month window period.

'Have you ever had sexual contact with another man/woman?' Record the response as part of your risk assessment if it hasn't been disclosed in the sexual history.

'*Have you ever had viral hepatitis?*' Record yes/no. If yes – which, A, B, C, etc. Any follow-up checks, treatment, etc.

'*Have you been vaccinated for hepatitis?*' Record yes/no. If yes – which, A, B, C, etc., and when completed. Any follow-up titre checks, etc.?

The questions in the following section are not currently routinely asked in the UK; however, asking them is common practice in the Australian and New Zealand sexual health services.

'*Have you ever "worked"?*' – If the person, usually female, has been a sex worker they will know what you are referring to – if they say, 'Yes, at Boots', you know that they are not likely to have been a sex-worker. Many people do not realise or forget that men too work in the sex industry. You don't need to pursue this point.

If yes, is the work current or previous. If current, continue with the following:

'*How many shifts a week?*' Record what you are told.

'*Any split or broken condoms (how many?) with customers?*' Record what is described. You should always re-establish that contraception is adequate. Sex workers often use condoms with customers but not with partners.

It is important to ensure that the worker is aware of the need for hepatitis vaccination, against both A and B, if they are continuing to work in the sex industry. Check if they are aware of the support workers in the community. You would need to know who the key workers are and how to contact them to make a referral.

HIV TESTING

'*Have you ever had an HIV test?*' Record yes/no, when and the result: this helps with the risk assessment if another test is to be done at this visit.

'*Would you be interested in having an HIV test today, as it is now a routine part of the STI screen?*' Record yes or no.

In many clinics at this point the history-taking would be terminated and the next phase of the process would be the examination. But increasingly the primary worker would continue and undertake the pre-HIV test discussion if the person is deemed to be low-risk and they are comfortable to continue. Most of the assessment questions have already been asked, so that now they need only cover the technical and legal aspects of the testing process.

You now perhaps have enough information to make a provisional diagnosis; however, until you complete the physical examination and collect the specimens you must keep your suspicions to yourself. It is important not to be drawn into making a diagnosis. If pressured you can use phrases such as '*It appears suggestive of X or Y; however, until the tests are done there is no definite answer.*'

This process is obviously a comprehensive breakdown of a sexual history-taking process. Many people are worried just how long this will take. In an asymptomatic person and with an experienced healthcare worker you may be able to complete this in 5 to 10 minutes maximum. Obviously every person should be treated in an individual manner, and therefore the time will vary.

To break down the process into a simpler form the following questions are a useful assessment guide.

The nature and duration of any symptoms.
When was the last time they had sex – was it within the last three months?
Describe the type of sex.
Were condoms used?
Do they know if the partner has symptoms?
Have they tried any self-medication to alleviate the symptoms?
Relevant medical history.
Medication allergies.
Current medication.
For women – the last menstrual period.

PREPARING FOR THE PHYSICAL EXAMINATION AND COLLECTION OF SPECIMENS

The next step should be to explain the examination process and the components of a basic sexual health screening available at your clinic/surgery/unit. Consent must be obtained before undertaking any form of intimate examination. This is achieved by explaining in full the procedure and the rationale for the investigations that may be carried out. This also allows the person time to raise any issues, worries or doubts that they may have. This is another time when cultural competence must be assessed: should a worker of the opposite gender to you undertake the examination?

As a practitioner you must be cognisant of this and offer a worker of the person's choice. Privacy and dignity must be ensured throughout the entire examination procedure. You must have explained what is going to happen and why prior to commencing. Many people feel vulnerable being undressed, and you should therefore keep the time they are undressed to an absolute minimum, providing where appropriate a blanket or disposable sheet to cover any exposed area before and during the examination (Randall et al., 1999; Torrance et al., 1999; Bignell, 1999).

It is strongly recommended now that all examinations regardless of the gender of the client/worker should be conducted in the presence of a chaperone. In some clinical areas this may be a friend or another healthcare worker. In some centres clients are asked whether they would like a chaperone present. At all times be guided by your local policies and the needs of your client and the staff (Clutterbuck, 2004).

REFERENCES

Barone M, Becker J (1999) Self-Instructional Module: STI's, HIV/AIDS, and Sexuality EngenderHealth. http://www.engenderhealth.org/res/onc/sexuality/talking/index. html accessed 19/09/2004

Bell HR (1998) *Men's Business, Women's Business: The Spiritual Role of Gender in the World's Oldest Culture.* Inner Traditions, Rochester, VT

Bignell CJ (1999) Chaperones for genital examination: Provide comfort and support for the patient and protection for the doctor. *British Medical Journal* 319 (7203) 137–8 (17 July)

Clutterbuck D (2004) *Sexually Transmitted Infections and HIV.* Elsevier Mosby, Edinburgh

Evans D (2004) Behind the headlines: sexual health implications for nursing ethics and practice. *Primary Health Care* Vol. 14 40–9

Fieldhouse R (2005) Snorting Coke and Hepatitis C http://www.ukcoalition.org/hepc/coke.htm accessed 01/09/05

Green J (1999) Taking a sexual history. *Trends in Urology Gynaecology and Sexual Health* September/October 31–3

Jones R, Barton S (2004) Introduction to History Taking and principles of sexual health. *Postgraduate Medical Journal* Vol. 80 444–6

Kurtz SM, Silverman JD, Draper J (1998) *Teaching and Learning Communication Skills in Medicine.* Radcliffe Medical Press, Oxford

Kurtz S, Silverman J, Benson J, Draper J (2003) Marrying Content and Process in Clinical Method Teaching: Enhancing the Calgary–Cambridge Guides. *Academic Medicine* Vol. 78 (8) 802–9

Law C, McCoriston P (1996) Taking a sexual history as part of the risk assessment for HIV & STDs. A guide for healthcare professionals (Video: 21.25 mins). St George's Hospital, Kogarah, Australia

Meacher P (1999) Inclusive questions are needed when taking a sexual history. *British Medical Journal* Vol. 318 1289

Potter J, Flory J (2004) Taking a Sexual History. Harvard Medical School Cultural Competence in Women's Health. http://www.hmcnet.harvard.edu/coe/cultural/html/repro-history.html accessed 19/09/2004

Presswell N, Barton D (2000) Taking a Sexual History. *Australian Family Physician* Vol. 6 (June 29) 535–9

Randall S, Webb A, Kishen M (1999) Chaperones for genital examination: Presence of chaperone may interfere with doctor–patient relationship. *British Medical Journal* 319(7219) 1266 (6 November)

Temple-Smith MJ, Mulvey G, Keogh L (1998) Attitudes to taking a sexual history in general practice in Victoria, Australia. *Sexually Transmitted Infections* Vol. 75 41–4

Tomlinson J (1998) ABC of sexual health. *British Medical Journal* Vol. 317 1573–6 (5 December)

Torrance CJ, Das R, Allison MC (1999) Use of chaperones in clinics for genitourinary medicine: survey of consultants. *British Medical Journal* Vol. 319(7203) 159–60 (17 July)

Verhoeven V, Bovijn K, Helder A, Peremans L, Hermann I, Van Royen P, Denekens J, Avonts D (2003) Discussing STI's: doctors are from Mars, patients are from Venus. *Family Practice* Vol. 20 (1) 11–15

3 Male Genital Examination

YASWANT (RAVI) DASS

INTRODUCTION

Examination of the male genital tract is essential in the diagnosis of sexually transmitted infections and for the differential diagnosis of such conditions. There are a number of different approaches that can be taken to conducting such an examination, but the main objective is to examine all the relevant anatomy. Sexually transmitted infections commonly affect other parts of the body, and examination of other systems/anatomy in addition to the male genital tract may be required (Barkauskas *et al.*, 2002), for example rectal examination; these are discussed in other chapters.

CONSENT AND CHAPERONING

Genital examination should never start without obtaining the patient's consent. It is essential to explain to the patient why the examination is necessary (Walsh *et al.*, 1999; Fuller & Schaller-Ayers, 2000) and how it will be conducted, and to reassure patients that it is non-invasive and should not hurt. This will ensure that verbal consent is obtained. Verbal or implied consent is sufficient, and written consent is not required for a genital examination. A further examination of issues of consent can be found in the chapter on Legal Issues.

Patients should be allowed to prepare for the examination by removing any clothing or underwear. This would imply that the patient is agreeing to be examined. The nurse must never undress the patient, unless in exceptional circumstances such as disability, when undressing the patient for genital examination must be done in the presence of a chaperone.

The clinician must always offer the patient a chaperone (Epstein *et al.*, 2000), and this must be clearly documented. If a chaperone is used, their name and designation must also be documented. Local policies regarding chaperoning vary, so always follow such policies, remembering that young men (under the age of 16) and those with disabilities will require a chaperone in all cases.

Advanced Clinical Skills for GU Nurses. Edited by Matthew Grundy-Bowers and Jonathan Davies
© 2007 John Wiley & Sons Ltd

MAINTAINING DIGNITY

Examination of the male genital tract needs to be conducted in a sensitive manner, and in privacy. Ensure that privacy can be maintained by locking doors, as this will prevent interruption from a third party and may also help to reassure patients. The examination room also needs to be adequately heated, because if the room is too cold the scrotal sack may contract and it may be more difficult to examine the scrotal contents.

Embarrassment is common during a genital examination (Toghill, 1994), and depending on the experience of the practitioner this procedure may cause some embarrassment for both practitioner and client. If the nurse appears nervous or embarrassed, the patient may well pick up on this and may become anxious or embarrassed too. It is always good practice to maintain conversation whilst conducting the examination, as this may help to distract clients or divert their attention. Talking about testicular cancer and testicular self-examination is always a suitable topic to engage clients with whilst conducting a genital tract examination.

Men with no previous experience of such a procedure may become aroused (Swartz, 2002), especially younger men, and it is essential that the nurse does not become embarrassed by this and offers reassurance to the client that such arousal is perfectly normal. The nurse should then complete the examination as quickly as possible and allow the patient to get dressed (Barkauskas et al., 2002).

On rare occasions some patients may try to cause embarrassment for the nurse through sexual comments or displaying sexual behaviour towards the health professional. This may be an intentional act on the part of the patient, or more often a manifestation of their nervousness or embarrassment. In these circumstances, a chaperone may be useful, and the nurse must remember to maintain professional boundaries. It is important in these circumstances to employ your clinical and professional judgement when assessing the situation. The use of gloves in all circumstances (Fuller & Schaller-Ayers, 2000) also emphasises the clinical nature of the examination (Epstein et al., 2000).

GROIN AND PUBIC AREA

INGUINAL LYMPH NODES

Literature supports the examination of the male patient in both the supine (Epstein et al., 2000; Swartz, 2002) and the standing position (Walsh et al., 1999; Fuller & Schaller-Ayers, 2000). The exceptional case for not laying the patient down is when checking for scrotal hernias and varicoceles. In a standing position the groin or inguinal area should be examined for lymphadenopath (enlargement of lymph nodes and also noting any tenderness). Even in the absence of any sexually transmitted infections, it may be possible to feel lymph nodes that may be non-tender and feel smooth like marbles. Normal lymph nodes can be up to 25 mm or 1 inch in length, so that the mere presence of palpable lymph nodes does not mean that they are abnormal. The lymph nodes are part of the lymphatic system (immune system), and their main function is to filter lymph fluid containing foreign particles, infective agents and malignant cells, as well as facilitating lymphocytes (white blood cells) in producing antibodies (killer cells) against invading organisms.

Lymph nodes may suddenly become swollen and tender as a result of infection or injury (Barkauskas *et al.*, 2002; Swartz, 2002), whereas gradual enlargement without tenderness may result from malignant changes. Patients with painless enlarged lymph nodes should be advised to see their general practitioner for a health check to investigate any systemic diseases. Most sexually transmitted infections (commonly HIV, syphilis, LGV and HSV) can cause acute enlargement and tenderness of lymph nodes. Infection of the genital tract would generally cause enlargement of the local inguinal lymph nodes, and once the infection has been treated the lymph nodes should return to normal in several weeks.

THE PUBIC SKIN

In order to undertake a thorough examination of skin in the genital area it is essential to use a good light with magnification (Fuller & Schaller-Ayers, 2000). The pubic area needs to be checked for infestations, molluscum contagiosum, genital warts, ulceration, dermatosis etc. It is possible to see *Phthirus pubis* (pubic lice) on pubic hairs or attached to the skin. These can be easily removed and placed on a microscopy slide for microscopic observation. The eggs of the pubic lice can also be seen adhering to the pubic hairs. Infestation with *Sarcoptes scabiei* (scabies) mites can commonly be seen in the pubic region, where papular skin eruptions emerge over burrows made by the egg-laying female mites. Both pubic lice and scabies infestation can cause intense pruritus, and evidence of scratching may be visible on the skin. Molluscum contagiosum and genital warts are commonly diagnosed by visual examination of the genital and pubic skin. Small white or skin-coloured dome-shaped papules, which are characteristic of molluscum contagiosum, and benign epidermal proliferations, ranging from flat keratinised to pedunculated fleshy warts, can be seen on the skin.

Multiple fluid-filled vesicles or painful ulcers may indicate infection with the *Herpes simplex* virus or chancroid, whereas a solitary painless ulcer with indurated margins may help the nurse to investigate primary syphilis infection or lymphogranuloma venereum.

Large areas of demarcated macular erythema may indicate a fungal infection such as *Tinea cruris* (jock itch). This can be easily treated with topical anti-fungal creams but the nurse should instruct the patient on appropriate hygiene requirements to ensure eradication. Erythema of the pubic skin may also result from other dermatological conditions such as eczema, psoriasis, etc., and patients should be advised to see a general practitioner/dermatologist for the management of any non-sexual skin condition.

PENIS

Ideally the penis should be examined prior to the client voiding urine, as this will reveal any apparent discharge. At this point the nurse can observe the penis for any abnormal curvature, such as those seen in Peyronie's Disease (Swartz, 2002). This is where internal scarring of the corpora cavernosa causes the penis to bend sharply up, down or to the side. Men with Peyronie's may experience pain during sexual intercourse, and, if the condition persists, they may eventually notice shortening of the penis, both of which can be distressing for the patients (Gholami and Lue, 2001). The exact cause of Peyronie's disease is uncertain, but it is probably caused by minor trauma to the penis, which leads to hardening of the tissue (fibrosis) of the tunica albuginea layer that surrounds the corpora cavernosa. The penis will bend in the direction of the fibrous scar tissue, so that if there is hardening on the right side of the penis then the penis will bend sharply right. Usually if the penis is palpated the hardened tissue can be felt. If Peyronie's Disease is suspected the nurse should then advise the patient to see his General Practitioner for a review and surgical referral.

The penile skin often contains visible Fordyce glands, which are sebaceous (fat-producing) glands (Swartz, 2002) to keep the penile skin lubricated. They can be easily mistaken for genital warts or molluscum contagiosum, despite being little fatty lumps under the skin. The sebaceous glands can become blocked or form into sebaceous cysts, and rarely may become infected. The patient needs to be reassured about their presence.

The prepuce (foreskin) if present, needs to be retracted, noting any phimosis (inability to retract the foreskin) (Swartz, 2002; Fuller & Schaller-Ayers, 2000). The examiner may want to retract the foreskin to determine its mobility (Swartz, 2002). Once the foreskin is retracted the glans penis and sub-prepuce skin can also be examined. It is important to note the presence of smegma (Swartz, 2002; Bellack & Edlund, 1992) or odour (Epstein *et al.*, 2000). It is common to find mild erythema of the prepuce, especially after sex or if proper hygiene care is not taken.

Inflammation of the glans penis (balanitis) and involving the prepuce (balano-posthitis) can be seen once the foreskin is retracted. Balanitis often results from poor hygiene, chemical irritants, bacterial or fungal infection, and drug allergies (sulfphonamides and tetracyclines), and is usually more commonly seen in uncircumcised men (Edwards, 1996). Often the inflamed skin has patches of erosion and linear fissuring can be seen especially on the foreskin. Fungal and bacterial causes should be investigated and balanitis should be treated, as the damaged skin poses a risk for acquiring infections.

Around the rim of the glans penis (corona) it is possible to see penile pearly papules. These are tiny filiform (thread-like) projections, which may range from being skin-coloured to white in colour, and are more common in uncircumcised men. Also located symmetrically either side of the frenulum are Tyson's glands. These are secretory glands that produce an oily substance to lubricate the prepuce. The nurse must reassure the patient that these are normal and not contagious and do not require treatment.

Using a thumb and forefinger, expose the external meatus (Fuller & Schaller-Ayers, 2000; Epstein *et al.*, 2000). The meatus is then located and the position noted, as sometimes the meatus may open on the underside or ventral side (hypospadias) (Epstein *et al.*, 2000) or on the upper surface or dorsum of the glans penis (epispadias). Some men may also present with multiple meatal openings; but usually only one is connected to the urethra. Spontaneous discharge can be detected from outside the meatus; but it is essential to part the meatus opening gently and check for meatal stenosis, ulceration, inflammation or warts. After being retracted, the foreskin should always be put back in its correct position to prevent paraphimosis (Swartz, 2002).

SCROTUM AND CONTENTS

The scrotal skin should be examined all the way down to the perineum. If the patient complains about symptoms on the scrotum/perineum it may be better to lay the patient's down for the examination. It is important to observe the patient's face during the examination to check for signs of discomfort (Epstein *et al.*, 2000).

Sebaceous cysts and angiokeratomas are often seen on the scrotal skin. Angiokeratomas appear as black, blue or dark red papules on the skin and they result from dilated capillaries in the dermis, which is covered by epidermal hyperplasia. Angiokeratomas may bleed as a result of friction during sexual intercourse, and may cause anxiety for the patient. Patients need to be reassured that they are not harmful, and that they can see a dermatologist for removal if so desired, although this procedure is not routinely performed.

The testes should be examined, noting any cryptorchidism (undescended testicle), differences in size of testicles, discomfort on exam, fluid collection or nodular growths. It is common for one testicle (usually the left) to hang slightly lower than the other testicle (Epstein *et al.*, 2000; Swartz, 2002), and if only one testicle is present it is important to get an accurate account of what happened to the other testicle. Using both hands the surface of each testicle needs to be palpated under the skin. Any lumps or gritty areas on a testicle (Fuller & Schaller-Ayers, 2000) or any unilateral enlargement should be further investigated with an ultrasound scan. Testicular cancer is a concern for men under the age of 40 and usually more common amongst men with a history of undescended testicles (Forman *et al.*, 1994). Patients with unde-scended testicles should be advised to see their general practitioner for surgi-cal referral, owing to the increased risk of testicular cancer. Information should be given to the patient regarding regular testicular self-examination at home (Walsh *et al.*, 1999).

The epididymis and vas deferens (spermatic cord) also need to be gently palpated (Swartz, 2002). Pain/tenderness with swelling of the epididymis or spermatic cord may indicate the presence of a descended infection. Epi-didymitis is most commonly caused by infections, and acute epididymitis may result in severe scrotal pain and swelling, so that it may be too painful to examine the scrotal contents at that point. Antibiotic treatment, analgesia (with an oral anti-inflammatory such as Ibuprofen) and scrotal support would usually resolve acute epididymitis.

The testicles can also twist on the spermatic cord (testicular torsion) result-ing in obstructed venous flow, pain, and swelling. This is a surgical emergency, as ischaemia can result in a loss of the testicle. If torsion is suspected the patient must be referred to the surgeons for immediate assessment.

Cysts often form in the comma-shaped epididymis, which is attached to the posterior of the testicle (Epstein *et al.*, 2000). Epididymal cysts contain fluids and may be multiple and/or bilateral and cause discomfort. On examination it is possible to palpate above the cysts, and they can be palpated separately from the testicles; they are also fluctuant (a wave-like motion is felt when they are palpated, owing to their containing fluid) and transilluminate (light up brightly when a light is pointed at the cyst in a darkened room). Men with asymptomatic epididymal cysts only require reassurance; but if they are uncomfortable, fluid from the epididymal cysts can be aspirated or they can be removed surgically. These treatment options are only performed after a man has no desire for further children, as scarring is possible after surgery/aspiration and this may cause blockage to the flow of sperm, resulting in infertility.

Infections and injury can lead to the formation of a hydrocele – a collection of serous fluid in the tunica vaginalis. Hydroceles are usually asymptomatic, transilluminate and can resolve without surgical intervention. The patient can visit his GP for further ultrasound scanning if still concerned.

Varicoceles can also be felt in the scrotal sac, and are often desribed as a sack of worms or spaghetti (Fuller & Schaller-Ayers, 2000). They are an enlarged mass of veins that develop in the spermatic cord when valves that regulate the flow of blood become defective, causing impaired circulation of blood away from the testicle and dilation of the veins. Varicoceles are more common on the left spermatic cord and are associated with infertility (Evers and Collins, 2003).

In clinical areas nurses can do a simple transillumination examination by placing the patient in a dark room and applying a strong light to the posterior testicle. The light will transmit through fluid-filled structures (hydroceles,

Table 2

Area	Findings
Lymph nodes	**Normal:** No lymphadenopathy or palpable shotty lymph nodes. **Abnormal:** Enlarged (put approximate size, e.g. 3 cm × 4 cm), state site (bilateral, left or right), pain or tenderness, hard or fluctuant.
Pubic/Genital skin	**Normal:** No abnormalities detected (NAD) **Abnormal:** Record findings such as warts, infestations, molluscum, ulceration, rashes, etc. and give a description: *Warts:* Number visible, location, flat keratinised/fleshy pedunculated *Rashes:* size and location of area, macular. Papular, diffused, circumscribed, appearance (inflammation, silvery surface, intact skin, exudation, dry, etc.). *Ulceration:* number, size, location, tenderness and appearance (superficial, skin erosion, indurated).
Penis	**Normal:** No abnormalities detected (NAD), circumcised or uncircumcised **Abnormal:** Record findings such as warts, infestations, molluscum, ulceration, rashes etc and give a description. *Meatus:* record any visible finding for meatal opening, such as discharge, inflammation, ulceration.
Scrotal contents	**Normal:** No abnormalities detected (NAD) **Abnormal:** *Testes:* Number present, abnormal sizes between the two, palpable lesion and location (posterior, anterior, superior, etc.), tenderness. *Epididymis:* swelling (cysts) or enlargement, lesions, tenderness, unilateral or bilateral. *Spermatic cord:* same as for epididymis

epididymal cysts, spermatoceles) and the structure will glow. However, light will not transmit though solid mass lesions, and these should be further investigated with ultrasound scanning if testicular malignancy is suspected (Krieger and Graney, 1999).

Essentially the lymph nodes, pubic skin, penis and scrotal contents need to be examined, and any findings must be clearly documented (see Table 2). It is always useful for abnormal findings to be drawn on a diagram of the male genital area. Most GUM clinics would have standard drawings for this purpose on either a proforma or a rubber stamp that can be used in the notes.

Examination of the male genitals may cause anxiety for the nurse starting to perform such examinations, but confidence comes with more experience. Essentially the lymph nodes, pubic skin, penis and scrotal contents need to be examined, and any findings to be clearly documented. This should be done as quickly as possible whilst maintaining the dignity of the patient. Providing adequate explanations for the procedure will secure the consent and co-operation of the patient and allow the nurse to conduct the examination in a very short time.

REFERENCES

Barkauskas VH, Baumann LC, Darling-Fisher CS (2002) *Health and Physical Assessment*, 3rd edn. Mosby, St Louis

Bellack J, Edlund C (1992) *Nursing Assessment and Diagnosis*, 2nd edn. Jones & Bartlett, Boston

Edwards, S (1996) Balanitis and balanoposthitis: a review. *Genitourinary Medicine* V 72 (3) 155–9

Epstein O, Perkin DG, de Bono DP, Cookson J (2000) *Clinical Examination*, 2nd edn. Mosby, St Louis

Evers JLH, Collins JA (2003) Assessment of efficacy of varicocele repair for male sub-fertility – a systematic review. *Lancet* V 361 (9372) 1849–52

Forman D, Pike MC, Davey G, Dawson S, Baker K, Chilvers CED, Oliver RTD, Coupland CAC (1994) Aetiology of testicular cancer: association with congenital abnormalities, age at puberty, infertility and exercise. *BMJ* V 308 (6941) 1393–9

Fuller J, Schaller-Ayers J (2000) *Health Assessment: A Nursing Approach*, 3rd edn. Lippincott, Philadelphia

Gholami SS, Lue TF (2001) Peyronie's disease. *Urologic Clinics of North America* V 28 (2) 377–90

Krieger JN, Graney DO (1999) Clinical anatomy, histology and physical examination of the male genital tract. In Holmes KK *et al. Sexually transmitted diseases*, 3rd edn. McGaw-Hill, New York

Swartz M (2002) *Textbook of Physical Assessment: History and Diagnosis*, 4th edn. Saunders, Philadelphia

Toghill P (1994) *Examining Patients: An Introduction to Clinical Medicine*, 2nd edn. Edward Arnold, London

Walsh M, Crumbie A, Reveley S (1999) *Nurse Practitioners: Clinical Skills and Professional Issues*. Butterworth Heinemann, Oxford

4 Female Genital Examination

MICHELLE ARNOLD

INTRODUCTION

Female genital examination and testing is essential to correct diagnosis and management of sexually transmitted infections in women. Developing a *rapport* with the client and maintaining her confidence throughout the examination is paramount, as some women may be fearful of the process, anticipating physical and psychological discomfort such as pain and embarrassment. Earlier negative experiences can exacerbate these fears. Although a means to effective examination, the speculum is not without emotive connotations for some women.

Establishing the woman's previous experience of examination, recognising and exploring any concerns and responding to verbal and non-verbal cues should be done prior to the woman's undressing for examination.

Verbal consent to examination should be obtained. The process and purpose of the examination should be fully explored to ensure that the consent that is given is truly informed. The patient should be advised to report any pain or discomfort experienced during the examination and that she can call a stop to the examination (i.e. consent can be withdrawn) at any time. In those under sixteen years, the Fraser guidelines (House of Lords, 1985) should be strictly adhered to in order to assess competence to consent to the examination. In Scotland, guidance is given in the form of The Age of Legal Capacity (Scotland) Act 1991. For further information see Chapter 7: Legal Issues in Sexual Health.

The use of a chaperone remains a grey area. A chaperone is one who observes the examination and can advocate on behalf of the client, supporting her during the procedure. As a witness to the examination, the chaperone may also advocate on behalf of the practitioner in the event of client complaint. Male practitioners have historically required a female chaperone during female examination. It is important that the chaperone is able to recognise, raise and justify concerns, possibly against a very senior colleague.

Advanced Clinical Skills for GU Nurses. Edited by Matthew Grundy-Bowers and Jonathan Davies
© 2007 John Wiley & Sons Ltd

An ineffective chaperone may be worse than no chaperone, as the client herself may be less likely to raise concerns or call a halt to the examination if the second person says nothing. In some cases an additional person in the examination room may exacerbate the woman's more general anxieties – for example, concerns about body image. Within current guidelines it is considered good practice to offer the client a chaperone; and it is essential in some circumstances. Clear documentation should be kept, including the name of the chaperone. Specific guidelines for nurses have been published by the Royal College of Nursing (RCN 2002).

MAINTAINING A SAFE ENVIRONMENT

Although female genital examination is not a sterile procedure, advance preparation of the clinical environment is necessary to maintain infection control during the examination. The examination couch is cleaned with detergent-based wipes and covered with examination paper. The examination trolley is cleaned with alcohol-based wipes and the examination light is cleaned also. Equipment is arranged so as to prevent possible cross-contamination during the procedure: for example, the light is positioned prior to the examination. Careful hand washing is necessary both before and immediately after the examination. Protective gloves should be worn during the procedure and when handling waste. Care should be taken to dispose of sharps and clinical or domestic waste appropriately.

Care should be taken to ensure correct labelling of all samples. Within GUM, samples are usually labelled with an individual clinic number and date of birth only. Details should be checked against the notes and confirmed with the patient.

It is important to confirm that the patient understands exactly which samples will (and will not) be taken. For example, clarification that a cervical smear is not part of the examination may influence her decision to attend for future cervical screening. On the basis of clinical findings, the need for additional samples may arise. The patient should be informed and give consent to all tests undertaken.

Privacy and dignity should be maintained at all times. The door should remain closed and curtains/screens should be used. The practitioner should leave the room to enable the woman to undress (from the waist down) in private. A cover should be offered and the patient invited to sit on the couch when changed. Before re-entering the room, the practitioner should knock and state his/her name.

It is important to ensure that the patient is correctly positioned on the couch and as comfortable as possible before starting the examination. The patient should be asked to sit at the front edge of the couch and then to lie back with the backs of the knees supported by the leg rests. Her arms should ideally rest at the side of her body, as stretching back tightens the abdominal muscles (Jarvis, 2000). Monitoring the patient during the examination (for example for gripping the couch or breath-holding) can enable feedback to be given to help reduce muscular tension, facilitating ease of examination for both patient and practitioner.

The practitioner should be aware of the potential risk of a vasovagal episode on taking cervical swabs. Assessment should be made to identify those prone to fainting, particularly women who have experienced a vasovagal episode during a previous examination. A colleague should be informed prior to the examination and emergency equipment (including oxygen) should be readily available. The patient should be observed for signs of pallor, yawning, dizziness, nausea or fainting during and immediately after the examination. After the examination, the practitioner should encourage the patient to remain supine and not to sit up too quickly.

THE EXAMINATION

INGUINAL LYMPH NODES

The nurse should warn the patient in advance of physical contact to ensure that the patient knows what to expect and when to expect it. The inguinal nodes in both groins should be gently palpated for swelling and the patient should be asked if there is any tenderness. Lymphadenopathy may be associated with infections such as *Herpes simplex* virus or syphilis.

EXTERNAL GENITAL EXAMINATION

The nurse should take a gentle but confident approach to the examination, examining all areas (including the outer labia majora and inner labia minora, the clitoral hood, the introitus, the pubic hair, the tops of the legs/buttocks, and perianal and anal areas) carefully and checking in skin folds. A dialogue should be maintained with the woman, with care taken to examine and feed back to her on any areas that she may be concerned about.

Pediculosis pubis

Pediculosis pubis (adult pubic lice and their eggs) can be found on the pubic and other body hair. These may have been transmitted during sexual or other close body contact. Lice and eggs can be removed gently from the hair or, with patient consent, scissors can be used to cut a small piece of the hair, for example with the egg *in situ*. It can then be placed on a slide under a cover slip and viewed in more detail under a light microscope.

Genital warts

External examination can reveal genital warts, painless growths that may be either soft and fleshy, with a typical 'cauliflower' appearance, or hard and keratinised. As genital warts are usually associated with low oncogenic risk human papilloma virus (HPV) types 6 and 11, women should be advised to continue routine cervical cytology.

Molluscum contagiosum

Molluscum contagiosum is caused by a pox virus, and appears as small white lesions, often with a characteristic umbilicated centre. Passed on easily through close physical contact, the lesions are commonly seen on the faces and arms of young children. In adults it is usually acquired through sexual contact, and lesions are found in the genital area or on the stomach and thighs.

Genital ulcers

Genital blisters or painful ulcers are most likely to typify *Herpes simplex* virus. With agreement from the patient, these can be sampled with a cotton-tipped swab and sent in medium to the laboratory for testing and possible typing. A painless solitary ulcer is most likely to typify a syphilitic chancre. Again in agreement with the patient, this should be scraped, and the serum collected on to a plain slide. A cover slip should be placed over the sample and it should be read for spirochetes on a dark-field microscope. Three samples should be taken at the first visit, and the sampling repeated over the next two days. Serological testing for syphilis should also be carried out at the first visit, although dark-field microscopy remains the test that will yield the earliest diagnosis. The tropical sexually transmitted infections, such as chancroid, lymphogranuloma venereum (LGV) and donovanosis are relatively uncommon in the UK, however, are important causes of genital ulcers in some regions of the world. Careful assessment prior to the examination, including recent travel history, should reveal if the patient has been at risk from partners in the areas where these conditions are endemic. Clinical signs alone cannot be relied upon to differentiate between the infective causes of genital ulcers; diagnostic testing is a vital component, as clinical manifestations do not always follow the textbook. Ulcerated areas may also be due to non-infective causes, such as scratching with vulvae pruritus or other physical trauma. Small blisters/ulcers may also be the 'satellite lesions' associated with the endogenous yeast infection, *Candida albicans*.

Bartholin's abscess

The ducts of Bartholin's glands open bilaterally at the introitus, and can become blocked and subsequently infected. As part of the examination, the site of the glands is observed for swelling and any reports of pain by the patient are elicited (Anderson *et al.*, 2005). Abscess formation can occur secondary to gonorrhoea or chlamydia; however, it is not always associated with a sexually transmitted organism. Bartholin's abscess should be observed for purulent discharge, and an additional swab sample obtained for microscopy culture and sensitivity (MC&S). If the abscess is non-discharging the patient will need to be referred directly to gynaecology for excision and drainage (Mitchell, 2004).

Genital dermatosis

Patients may also present with dermatological conditions, such as eczema and psoriasis. Symptoms manifest differently in the vulval area. Review by a dermatologist is necessary to ensure an accurate diagnosis. Any unusual growths, discoloration or pigmentation should be referred for prompt review and possible biopsy. These may be associated with vulval carcinomas or possible precursor disease, such as Bowen's.

Female circumcision

Although illegal in the United Kingdom, female circumcision (also known as female genital mutilation) is still practised within some cultures. This involves deliberate physical damage to the architecture of the vulva of the adolescent or young woman. It is usually carried out by older women within the same culture. The procedure may be carried out with or without anaesthesia; however, with anaesthesia the extent of the circumcision can be even more radical. Ill consequences to health include menstrual problems, recurrent urinary tract infections, pain and difficulties having sex, reduced sexual pleasure (from partial or complete removal of the clitoris) and obstructed labour (http://www.who.int/mediacentre/factsheets/fs241/en/index.html). Sensitivity in dealing with this complex issue is vital. Other young women in the same family or social network may be at future risk, and there may be an opportunity for intervention to prevent this.

SPECULUM EXAMINATION

A metal speculum should be warmed to body temperature prior to use; however, a plastic speculum can be used at room temperature. A small amount of water-based lubricant may be required to facilitate ease of examination and increased comfort for the woman. The patient should be advised as to expected sensations (for example, a stretching sensation on opening the blades). Non-verbal and verbal cues should be monitored carefully during the examination, and the pace of the examination should be adapted to the individual. Pausing at the introitus before passing the speculum allows for the patient to register the fact that the examination is about to begin at a physiological level. A gentle but confident approach should be taken. The speculum is passed slowly and smoothly, taking care not to trap the pubic hair or labia. Unless the uterus is known to be retroverted, the speculum is introduced according to the physiological tilt of the vagina (upwards at an approximately 45-degree angle). Once fully inserted, the blades are opened slightly, and if necessary minor adjustments are made until the cervix is in view. Once the cervix is visible, the blades can be opened further to bring the cervix fully into view. Care should be taken to avoid pressing against the urethra during the process of adjustment. If the uterus is retroverted, it may be necessary to remove and reposition the speculum accordingly.

Once the speculum is in place, careful observation should be made of the vagina and cervix. A sample may be taken from the lateral vaginal walls for *Candida* and bacterial vaginosis using either a cotton-tipped or a loop swab. To ensure a good sample, a scraping action to the actual walls of the vagina is used (as opposed to just collecting vaginal discharge). The sample is then applied thinly to a plain slide, in preparation for Gram stain and microscopy. The same sample may also be used to culture for *Candida*, for example, using the Saboraud medium. A gentle sweeping action should be used to ensure that the agar remains intact. Using the same type of swab a sample is taken from the posterior fornix (at the top of the vagina, underneath the cervix) for *Trichomonas vaginalis*. A sweeping motion from side to side is used. Once the sample has been obtained the swab is gently agitated into a few drops of normal (0.9%) saline on a plain slide and a cover slip is then applied. This 'wet prep' or 'wet mount' sample can be read in either a dark or light microscope for trichomonads.

In preparation for gonorrhoea and *Chlamydia* samples, a larger cotton-tipped swab or 'mop' is gently used to sweep away excess mucus from the cervix. Usually one mop is sufficient, but it is useful to have an extra one ready to hand for heavier cervical discharge/blood. The gonorrhoea sample is collected first, using the same type of swab as for vaginal samples. The tip of the swab is gently inserted into the cervical os. All aspects of the cervical opening should be fully sampled using a rotational movement and the swab removed. The sample can be applied thinly to a plain slide for Gram stain and microscopy and inoculated into a selective medium for culture and sensitivity tests on *Neisseria gonorrhoeae*. Again, a gentle sweeping action is used to ensure the agar remains intact. A cotton-tipped cervical swab is supplied with the appropriate *Chlamydia* testing kit. The tip of the swab is gently inserted into the cervical os and then agitated in a circular motion for at least 10 seconds or as per the manufacturer's instructions. To ensure a good specimen is collected all aspects of the cervical opening should be sampled and firm pressure used to pick up cervical cells. The sample is then placed into the *Chlamydia* transport medium.

VAGINAL EXAMINATION

Vaginal walls: a mucous discharge is normally present. This has a cleansing and protective function. The amount, colour and consistency of mucous discharge changes during the menstrual cycle and also with use of hormonal contraception. Typically there is a small–moderate amount of whitish discharge normally present. Observe for abnormal discharge, which may be caused by a non-sexually or a sexually acquired infection.

NON-SEXUALLY ACQUIRED CONDITIONS

Candida albicans

Candida albicans can have a watery or lumpy 'cottage cheese' type appearance and a 'yeasty' smell. There is usually intense itching/soreness, exacerbated by the itch/scratch cycle. In severe cases, this can impact on the activities of living and interfere with sleep. *Candida* is not a sexually transmitted infection (there is little/no benefit to treating asymptomatic partners), but is caused by an overgrowth of yeast organisms found commensally in the vagina. Diabetic and pregnant women are particularly susceptible; however, most women will experience at least one episode during their lifetimes.

Bacterial vaginosis

Bacterial vaginosis can be indicated if there is a grey/white thin, homogeneous discharge with a pungent, unpleasant 'fishy' odour. There may be a minimal amount of discharge coating the vaginal walls or copious amounts, which may be present on the vulva prior to examination or pour into the speculum on insertion. BV is not usually associated with vaginitis; however, there may be some physical irritation (such as itching) from the presence of the discharge. The discharge and associated odour can be particularly unpleasant and impact on self-esteem and relationships. The aetiology of BV is uncertain, but it is not considered to be a sexually transmitted infection, and there is little/no benefit in treating sexual partners. Over-zealous hygiene (including more than daily washing and washing inside the vagina), bathing in antiseptic solutions, bubble baths and washing the genital area with perfumed soaps and shower gels appear to exacerbate the problem. The infection is associated with an overgrowth of commensal bacteria and the loss of protective lactobacilli.

SEXUALLY ACQUIRED INFECTIONS

Changes in the normal vaginal discharge are a key symptom of sexually transmitted infection. Infective discharge may be mucopurulent, yellow-coloured with *Chlamydia* or purulent and greenish with gonorrhoea. The cervix can also appear red and inflamed, and there can be bleeding on contact with the swab. The woman may report bleeding after sex or between periods as a symptom.

Trichomonas vaginalis

Clinical signs of *Trichomonas* vaginalis include a frothy grey/green discharge at the posterior fornix. There may also classically be pedunculated red patches observable on the cervix. This is known as a 'strawberry cervix' by analogy with strawberry patches.

   Diagnosis should not rely on clinical signs alone, however, as these lack specificity; the use of a valid and reliable test that is sensitive and specific to a particular infection is essential to accurate and effective management. Careful swab technique (according to the manufacturer's instructions) and appropriate and timely storage and transfer of specimens ensure that this is maximised.

OTHER CAUSES OF VAGINAL DISCHARGE

Women with a cervical polyp may present with vaginal discharge, which may be brownish or bloodstained. On examination, polyps may be seen protruding from the cervical os. The woman should be referred to gynaecology for assessment and excision.

PHYSIOLOGICAL VARIATIONS

Cervical ectopy

A red appearance of the cervix is not necessarily pathological, but may be due to the outward movement of the transformation zone under the influence of high circulating levels of oestrogen, particularly in young women or those taking the combined oral contraceptive pill. The soft, mucus-producing columnar cells that usually line the endocervical canal are seen on the outside of the cervix: this is known as 'ectopy' or 'an ectropian', and is a normal physiological variation. For some women, however, it may be associated with increased physiological discharge or with contact bleeding (for example, after sex). Information should be given, which may provide reassurance; however, the discharge may be particularly heavy and problematic for some women (for example requiring frequent changes of sanitary protection). Although a normal variation, symptoms can sometimes be improved through treatment with cold coagulation, which (paradoxically) uses heat to the cervix to destroy the cells physically. Where ectopy is problematic, referral to colposcopy is necessary for appropriate assessment prior to treatment.

Nabothian follicles

Nabothian follicles may appear as small white papules on the cervix. These are not harmful and may eventually disappear.

CERVICAL CYTOLOGY

Routine cervical cytology is ideally carried out within general practice or community contraception clinics where follow-up of patients may be less problematic than within the GUM setting. However, there is a role for GUM practitioners in promoting understanding and allaying fears about the cervical screening programme, and in encouraging women to attend for smears. The history of cervical screening should be discussed and documented. Where the woman has missed attending for smears and is unlikely to attend other services, an opportunistic smear carried out with the woman's consent may be a pragmatic solution, and should be taken prior to cervical swabs to ensure an adequate sample. A smear should also be considered with clinical signs and symptoms, including unexplained bleeding and clinically abnormal changes to the cervix. An urgent referral should be made to colposcopy for further assessment.

REMOVING THE SPECULUM

Removing the speculum after the examination should be approached with as much care as insertion so as to avoid unnecessary discomfort. The speculum should be moved away from the cervix before beginning to close the blades. The blades are then closed smoothly and slowly and the speculum withdrawn, taking care to avoid trapping the vaginal walls, the labia or the pubic hair in the blades.

BIMANUAL EXAMINATION

During bimanual examination the practitioner gently inserts one or two gloved fingers into the vagina using water-based lubricant. The other hand is used to palpate across the abdomen. A gentle but firm approach is taken to feel the reproductive organs, checking for signs of tenderness/pain and any masses. Verbal and non-verbal communication should be closely monitored throughout the examination. A mass is highly likely to be a fibroid, although it could be a malignant tumour, and should be referred for further investigation. Within a GUM setting significant adnexal tenderness would be presumptively treated as Pelvic Inflammatory Disease (PID). If the fallopian tubes are palpable or pulsating ectopic pregnancy should be considered. In this event urgent referral to gynaecology is indicated (Jarvis, 2000).

After the examination tissues should be offered to remove the lubricant if any was used. It is important to pre-empt possible concerns; for example, the patient may experience light bleeding following cervical tests, which is normal. Sanitary protection should be offered if bleeding was noted on examination.

DOCUMENTATION

The examination findings should be clearly documented in the notes. Information should be included as to all aspects of the examination, with clear and meaningful descriptions and diagrams. All entries should be signed, and the name and designation of the practitioner clearly printed.

COMPETENCIES

The practitioner should work within his or her own limitations and competencies, seeking advice or referring a more complex case or difficult examination to a senior colleague if appropriate. Specialist competencies for sexual and reproductive health have been published by the RCN (2004) to give guidance to nurses at all levels.

REFERENCES

Anderson E, Gebbie A, Smith N, Berry P (2005) The Reproductive System. In Douglas G, Nicol F, Robertson C (eds), *Macleod's Clinical Examination*. Churchill-Livingstone, Edinburgh

Female Genital Mutilation fact sheet (2005) World Health Organization [online] Available from: http://www.who.int/mediacentre/factsheets/fs241/en/index.html [Accessed September 2005]

House of Lords (1985) Lords Fraser in the case of Gillick vs West Norfolk and Wisbech AHA and DHSS

Jarvis C (2000) *Physical Examination and Health Assessment*, 3rd edn. W. B. Saunders Company, Philadelphia

Mitchell H (2004) Other conditions that effect the female genital tract. In Adler M, Cowan F, French P, Mitchell H, Richens J (eds), *ABC of Sexually Transmitted Infections*. BMJ Books, London

RCN (Royal College of Nursing) (2002) *Chaperoning: The Role of the Nurse and the Rights of the Patient*. RCN, London

RCN (Royal College of Nursing) (2004) *Sexual Health Competencies: An Integrated Career and Competency Framework for Sexual and Reproductive Health Nursing*. RCN, London

5 The Skin and the Lymphatic System

JANE BICKFORD

INTRODUCTION

In this chapter the external genital examination will be considered. External genital examination is an important part of the procedure within genito-urinary medicine clinics. Its purpose is to examine and note the external genital anatomy, observe the skin for any anomalies and palpate the inguinal lymph nodes for evidence of swelling or tenderness. It should also be appreciated that this examination is intimate, and care should be taken to ensure that all procedures and their rationales are explained and consent is gained before the examination. It is good practice for medical staff to offer a chaperone for the intimate examination (GMC, 2001). There is currently no guidance for nursing staff regarding chaperones for intimate examination, but it is important to ensure the smooth running of the examination that both the patient *and* the nurse are comfortable and consent to the procedure. The examination should ideally take place in a well-lit location that is both private and free from interruption and as comfortable as possible for the patient. The examiner's comfort needs also to be considered, particularly in a busy clinic situation, where many patients will be examined by the same practitioner. The examination couch should be capable of mechanical manoeuvring to limit the amount of bending and stretching needed on the part of the examiner. The light source, equally, should be both adequate and movable. Female patients are most readily examined in the lithotomy position.

Examination of two major systems is involved in the external genital examination. These are the skin and the lymph systems. Additionally, genital anatomy is observed. In the following sections these three areas are considered, followed by a description of the more common anomalies seen in UK genito-urinary medicine (GUM) clinics.

Advanced Clinical Skills for GU Nurses. Edited by Matthew Grundy-Bowers and Jonathan Davies
© 2007 John Wiley & Sons Ltd

ANATOMY AND FUNCTION OF THE LYMPH SYSTEM

The lymphatic system is a network of vessels throughout the body. It is part of the body's immune system and is involved in the removal of foreign matter and cell debris. Lymph vessels are usually associated with the circulatory system, and lymph originates from lost blood plasma or interstitial fluid from the capillary beds. The lymph system serves to filter and return this fluid to the circulatory system.

The lymph organs are divided into primary and secondary organs. The bone marrow and the thymus belong to the primary organ category and the spleen, lymph nodes and secondary lymphoid tissues, such as the tonsils and the appendix, are known as the secondary lymph organs.

Lymphocytes are produced by stem cells in the bone marrow and either mature in the bone marrow (B lymphocytes) or the thymus (T lymphocytes). Both B and T lymphocytes circulate in the lymph and accumulate in the secondary lymph organs, waiting to encounter antigens such as micro-organisms.

The lymph nodes and organs function to filter and process other organisms or abnormal cells from the body. They are present in clusters in the armpits, on either side of the neck, in the chest, in the abdomen and in the groin. Lymph nodes have an internal honeycomb-like structure of connective tissue that is filled with lymphocytes. In the presence of infection the lymphocytes rapidly multiply, producing characteristic swelling and tenderness.

For the purposes of genital and pubic examination the inguinal lymph nodes should be gently palpated and any tenderness or swelling should be noted. Infective processes may lead to lymph-node enlargement; however, malignancy should also be considered if there is no other explanation for enlarged lymph nodes.

ANATOMY AND FUNCTION OF SKIN

Skin is the largest organ of the body and is our first barrier against harmful agents, biological or other. Skin is what keeps our internal environment balanced, and loss of skin integrity through burns, infection or injury can lead to massive dehydration. Temperature regulation, sensation, lubrication and body odour are all functions of skin. The skin is made up of three layers: the epidermis, the dermis and the basal layer. These are briefly considered below.

EPIDERMIS

The epidermis or outer layer of the skin is formed of keratinocytes. The outermost part of the epidermis is the horny layer (stratum corneum), and is formed of flattened dead keratinocytes. The epidermis consists of sub-layers of keratinocytes, which develop at the bottom and rise to the top, where they are eventually shed. Melanocytes and dendrititc cells are also found in the epidermis. Melanocytes, as their name suggests, are responsible for the production of melanin, and dendritic cells are part of the epidermal immune system.

DERMIS

The dermis is predominantly formed of connective tissue and is responsible for the skin's elasticity and strength. The dermis is vascular, and supplies nutrients to the avascular epidermis. It also contains hair follicles, sweat glands, sebaceous glands and nerve endings.

BASAL LAYER

This is the bottom layer of the skin, from which keratinocytes are formed.

ANATOMY AND EXAMINATION OF EXTERNAL GENITALIA

The genitalia of males and females do not differentiate until week seven of embryonic life. Undifferentiated genitalia consist of a phallus, which becomes either a glans penis or a clitoris, the labio-scrotal swelling, which becomes the scrotal sac or the labia majora, a urogenital fold and the urogenital membrane. The penis around the urethra in males equates to the labia minora in females.

The external genital examination for females involves examination of the mons pubis, the clitoris, the labia majora, and the labia minora along with the openings of the vagina and the introitus. For males the external structures are the penis, the prepuce if present and the scrotum and its contents. The prepuce in the male forms a covering of the glans penis and is also known as the foreskin; in the female the prepuce covers the clitoris and is also known as the clitoral hood. The prepuce of an uncircumcised man should be retracted to allow visual examination of the glans penis. Excision of both the male and the female prepuce occurs in certain cultures, and this is discussed below.

External examination requires good lighting. A magnifying glass is also a useful tool for the examination of small lesions. The skin is observed for presence of inflammation, excoriation, ulceration, integrity and pigmentation changes. Pubic hair is inspected for signs of infestation and the presence of any warts or other skin tumours is noted. Skin texture is inspected and any thickening or atrophy noted. The inguinal lymph nodes are palpated and swelling or discomfort noted. The contents of the scrotal sac are examined by palpation. The structures are identified and any pain, discomfort, thickening or abnormalities are noted.

ANATOMICAL ANOMALIES

MALE AND FEMALE CIRCUMCISION (FEMALE GENITAL MUTILATION OR FEMALE GENITAL CUTTING)

There are few medical conditions that require therapeutic male circumcision, and the British Association of Paediatric Surgeons/Royal College of Surgeons (2001) statement indicates that pathological phimosis is the one absolute medical indication. However, many men seen in UK GUM clinics are circumcised, a condition which results from the removal of the prepuce.

Female circumcision or female genital mutilation (FGM) or genital cutting is far less commonly seen. Strictly speaking 'circumcision' refers to the excision of the clitoral prepuce; however, this term, when applied to women, is often used to describe a number of different procedures involving alteration and removal of parts of the female genitalia. The term chosen by the World Health Organisation to describe these practices is female genital mutilation (FGM). I shall use this term; but practitioners should be aware that women who have undergone these procedures may refer to them as 'cutting' or 'circumcision'.

FGM has been illegal in the UK since the Prohibition of Female Circumcision Act was passed in 1985, and since 2004 it has also been illegal to take young girls abroad to have the procedure performed. About 74,000 women in the UK have had the procedure, and it has been estimated that about 7,000 girls under 17 are at risk (DfES 2004).

DEFINITION OF FGM

The two most common forms of mutilation are excision and infibulation.

Infibulation

Infibulation, also known as pharaonic circumcision, consists of clitoridectomy, excision of the labia minora, and cutting of the labia majora to create raw surfaces, which are then stitched or held together in order to form a cover over the vagina when they heal. A small hole is left to allow urine and menstrual blood to escape (Amnesty International, 2004).

Excision

Excision involves total or partial removal of the prepuce, clitoris and/or labia minora. Other mutilations include pricking, piercing or stretching of the clitoris and/or labia, cauterisation by burning of the clitoris and surrounding tissues, scraping of the vaginal orifice or cutting of the vagina, and introduction of corrosive substances into the vagina to cause bleeding or herbs into the vagina with the aim of tightening or narrowing it. Women who have undergone FGM often experience problems with their sexual, reproductive and general health. They may have difficulty with voiding or menstruating, and be prone to fistula and keloid formation, recurrent urinary tract infections or pelvic infections.

HYPOSPADIAS

Hypospadias is a congenital malformation that occurs in males. Hypospadias results in the urethral opening and meatus being located on the ventral penile surface. The consequence of hypospadias can be problems relating to the direction of urinary flow. These will be more or less severe depending on the location of the hypospadias. Examination of the penis will reveal hypospadias and, if the hypospadias is problematic, the adult male is usually aware of this.

SKIN ANOMALIES – NON-PATHOLOGICAL

FORDYCE SPOTS

Fordyce spots are ectopic sebaceous glands, and are seen primarily on the labia minora and the shaft of the penis. They are large sebaceous glands seen through mucosal skin. Their appearance is that of small yellow spots.

ANGIOKERATOMA

Angiokeratomas are more common in older people, and are tiny clusters of dilated blood vessels associated with keratinised tissue. They may be bright red, and will often darken to black with time. They are mainly seen on the scrotal skin in men and the labia majora in women.

VESTIBULAR PAPILLOMATOSIS

Vestibular papillomas are finger-like protrusions of the modified mucous membrane of the introitus and medial labia minora, and are sometimes mistaken for soft warts. Extensive studies of many individuals have not demonstrated the presence of HPV, and they are asymptomatic, requiring no treatment.

PEARLY PENILE PAPULES

Pearly penile papules are common dome-shaped papules that occur in rows around the coronal edge. They are more common in uncircumcised men, and their uniform, smooth appearance and arrangement in rows distinguish them from warts.

SKIN ANOMALIES – PATHOLOGICAL, NON-INFECTIVE

LICHEN SCLEROSIS

Lichen sclerosis is an inflammatory condition of unknown aetiology that most commonly occurs in the anogenital skin of both men and women. The main symptoms are itchiness and soreness; however, lichen sclerosis can occur without symptoms. Lichen sclerosis causes typical white plaques on the skin of the genitalia. Characteristic features in women are whitening and scarring atrophy, causing gradual destruction of normal vulval architecture, with burying of the clitoris and reabsorption of the labia minora. Eventual narrowing of the introitus is also known to occur. Lichen sclerosis may occur in skin already scarred or damaged (the Koebner phenomenon), so that trauma, injury, and sexual abuse have been suggested as possible triggers of symptoms in predisposed people. There is a small risk of developing squamous cell carcinoma on a background of lichen sclerosis, and biopsy of suspicious lesions is common.

LICHEN PLANUS

Lichen planus is an inflammatory eruption of the skin and mucous membranes of unknown aetiology. In the reticular (lacy) pattern there may be mild to severe pruritus, and the erosive and ulcerative form presents with pain and burning. On examination there may be small purple papules with a lacy or reticulated surface. In erosive disease there may be a glazed erythema with tenderness to touch or frank almost ulcerated erosions, often with a lacy or slightly greyish edge.

LICHEN SIMPLEX

Classically this condition is the end-result of intense, chronic pruritus that results from repetitive rubbing or scratching. The skin responds by thickening and the increase in skin markings is referred to as lichenification. This occurs mostly in individuals with a history of allergies, eczema, hay fever or asthma. They have sensitive and easily irritated skin.

VITILIGO

Vitiligo is thought to be an autoimmune disease in which the melanocytes at the border of the dermis and epidermis are destroyed. It tends to occur around orifices, and genital skin involvement sometimes occurs before involvement of other parts of the body. It is characterised by patches of sharply demarcated milk white skin with no signs of texture change.

ECZEMA

Eczema is a non-infectious condition that may develop following skin irritation or via an immune pathway. Eczema is a collection of clinical findings rather than a particular disease. Patients may present with papules, vesicles, erythema, fissures, weeping and oedema in an acute stage. Itching is often present, and angular and linear erosions produced by finger nails are common. Scaling and lichenification are common in the chronic stage. When lichenification occurs on the mucous membrane of the vulva the skin frequently becomes white.

PSORIASIS

Psoriasis often affects the genital area and typically presents as a well-demarcated pink plaque. The glans penis is a common site, and psoriasis of the vulva can present as discomfort. Other mucosal sites are rarely affected. Because of the moist nature of the genitalia the scaly nature of psoriasis is not readily obvious in psoriasis of the genitalia compared with that of other parts of the body.

CONTACT DERMATITIS

Contact dermatitis of the genital skin falls into two categories: irritant contact dermatitis and allergic contact dermatitis. Irritant contact dermatitis is a response to contact with an irritating substance. This is considered a mild chemical burn, and the appearance is erythematous, with oedema and exudation in more severe cases. It occurs rapidly, and is treated by elimination of the irritant. Allergic contact dermatitis occurs more slowly following contact with an allergen, and appears more like eczema, though allergic and irritant contact dermatitis are frequently indistinguishable.

PATHOLOGICAL INFECTIVE SKIN 'RASHES' THAT MAY BE SEEN IN GUM CLINICS

SECONDARY SYPHILIS

Lesions associated with secondary or disseminated syphilis occur more than three weeks, and usually four to ten weeks, following initial inoculation with *Treponema pallidum*. The rash of secondary syphilis is reported to start as an evanescent macular rash that usually goes unnoticed by both patient and clinician. A few days later a symmetrical papular eruption appears that involves the whole trunk and the extremities, including the palms of the hands and the soles of the feet. Papules are typically red or reddish brown, discrete, and 0.5–1.0 cm in diameter. Usually scaly, they may also be smooth, follicular or pustular (Musher, cited in Holmes *et al.* 1999).

HIV SERO-CONVERSION

The skin rash associated with HIV sero-conversion is described as red and macular, suggestive of pityriasis rosea, but extending to the face and the palms of the hand and soles of the feet (Hawkins cited in Gazzard, 2002).

FUNGAL INFECTIONS

Candida infections

Candida infections can cause marked skin irritation and oedema. Erythema is commonly present in women and fissuring may occur at the introitus. Though infection is less common in men, mild erythema and balanitis or balanoposthitis may occur, with fissuring of the prepuce.

Tinea cruris

Tinea cruris is a fungal infection that occurs mainly in the groin of adult men. The rash has a scaly raised red border that spreads down the inner thighs from the groin or scrotum. It may form ring-like patterns and is similar to tinea corporis or ringworm. It is not often seen on the penis or vulva or around the anus.

GENITAL WARTS

Genital warts are caused by human papillomavirus (HPV). Those with genital warts usually report the appearance of lumps or growths on their genitalia. Occasionally other symptoms such as itchiness are reported. A diagnosis of genital warts is made by visualisation of the lesions. Genital warts usually appear in women at the introitus, vulva, perineum and perianal area, and in men on the penis, scrotum, urethral meatus and perianal area. It is less common to find them on the vaginal walls or cervix in women. Areas of friction during sex are more commonly associated with warts.

Different morphologies exist: condylomata acuminata are cauliflower-like peduculated warts that are skin-coloured; warts may also be flat or dome-shaped. However, despite differing appearances most genital warts are caused by HPV type 6 or 11. Differential diagnoses include the condylomata lata of secondary syphilis and tumours either malignant or benign.

CONDYLOMATA LATA

Condylomata lata occur in a small proportion of patients with secondary syphilis. The lesions are moist, wart-like lesions that are highly infectious. They tend to present in moist, warm areas, and are generally whitish or grey.

GENITAL ULCER DISEASES

Most sexually transmitted genital ulcers in the UK are caused by *Herpes simplex* virus (HPA, 2005). *Treponema pallidum* is another common cause. Dark-ground microscopy, serological testing for syphilis and *Herpes simplex* culture can be performed to aid diagnosis. Nucleic acid amplification tests are also available for both organisms. Other sexually transmitted infective causes such as lymphogranuloma venereum, *Haemophilus ducreyi* and donovanosis should be considered, and a good travel history of both the patient and their partners is helpful. Other non-infective causes of genital ulcer disease include Behçet's disease and Crohn's disease.

HERPES SIMPLEX VIRUS

Herpes simplex virus typically presents as multiple painful vesicles or pustules, which break down to form erosive ulcers. These are generally painful and may coalesce to form larger areas of painful ulceration. True primary episodes are generally more severe than subsequent episodes, and are often associated with systemic symptoms. Many people, however, are unaware they are infected, as they do not experience symptoms. Asymptomatic shedding of *Herpes simplex* virus has been shown to occur and is probably an important means of transmission. An understanding of asymptomatic shedding can facilitate acceptance of what may become a chronic recurring condition. Differential diagnoses include primary syphilis, candidiasis, contact dermatitis and fixed drug reaction.

PRIMARY CHANCRE

The ulcer of primary syphilis (chancre) occurs 14 to 21 days following exposure. A painless papule appears at the site of inoculation. This grows to 0.5 to 1.5 cm, ulcerates and becomes a chancre (Musher, cited in Holmes, 1999). The chancre of primary syphilis is typically a single, painless ulcer with an indurated margin and a clean base. However, they may also be multiple, painful, purulent and destructive (BASHH, 2002). They occur typically in the genital, perineal or anal area and are associated with inguinal lymphadenopathy. Any part of the body can, however, be affected, and oral lesions are not uncommon if oral sex has occurred.

Genital lesions are typically seen on the penis of men and the labia, fourchette or cervix of women. Chancres of the anus or rectum also occur. Thorough sexual history-taking will lead to appropriate physical examination and subsequent observation of lesions. Dark-ground microscopy can be performed to visualise *Treponema pallidum*, though this should not be attempted from oral lesions to avoid confusion with a similar non-pathogenic organism that may be found in the mouth. Syphilis serology should be performed and repeated at three months if negative.

TROPICAL ULCERS

LYMPHOGRANULOMA VENEREUM (LGV)

LGV is caused by one of the serovars (L1, L2 or L3) of *Chlamydia trachomatis*. The primary skin lesion may well go unnoticed, and is described as a painless papule, pustule or erosion. These organisms are lymphotropic and, in the secondary phase, the main symptoms of LGV are associated with the lymph nodes. The most common sign is tender inguinal and/or femoral lymphadenopathy. Buboes may form and there may be chronic ulceration and fistula formation. Acute haemorrhagic proctitis may also occur. Since 2003 a series of outbreaks of LGV have been reported in European cities (HPA, 2005). These have been among men who have sex with men (MSM), and most cases present with proctitis.

CHANCROID (*HAEMOPHILUS DUCREYI*)

Chancroid usually presents as single or multiple soft sores that are painful and bleed easily. The base is necrotic and the borders ragged. Painful inguinal adenitis is common, and buboes develop that may rupture and result in extensive ulceration.

DONOVANOSIS OR GRANULOMA INGUINALE (*KLEBSIELLA GRANULOMATIS*)

Donovanosis presents with one or more papules or nodules that develop into friable ulcers that gradually increase in size. Lesions tend to be painless. Lymph nodes swell and infection may spread to tissue above the lymph nodes, leading to an abscess known as a psuedo-bubo or to skin ulceration.

OTHER INFECTIVE CONDITIONS COMMONLY SEEN IN GUM CLINICS

MOLLUSCUM CONTAGIOSUM

Caused by the molluscum contagiosum virus (MCV) which is a member of the pox virus family. The incubation period for MCV is usually 2–3 months. MCV produces flesh-coloured papules which grow over several weeks to a diameter of 3–5 mm. They are smooth, firm and dome-shaped, with a characteristic central umbilication. Occasionally they can grow to 10–15 mm (giant molluscum). Papules generally appear on the thighs, the buttocks, the inguinal region and occasionally the lower abdomen. They are less commonly found on the external genitalia or the perianal area.

PUBIC LICE

Adult lice and their eggs can be seen with the naked eye and may appear initially as scabs. Closer visualisation using magnification reveals their true identity. The insects feed on host blood, which they obtain by biting. Patients may present with itching or redness, which is a result of the bites. This reaction varies from person to person. Generally in unexposed people a period of five days can pass before allergic sensitisation occurs, leading to itching, which in turn leads to scratching, erythema, and inflammation. It may be possible also to observe dark-coloured specks on the skin or underwear. There are louse excreta.

REFERENCES

Amnesty International (2004) Female Genital Mutilation. www.amnesty.org.uk, accessed 23/08/2006

BASHH (British Association for Sexual Health and HIV) (2002) UK National Guidelines on the Management of Early Syphilis. www.bashh.org, accessed 26/02/2006

British Association of Paediatric Surgeons (2001) Press release RCS 2001, www.baps.org.uk, accessed 25/02/2006

DfES (Department for Education and Skills) (2004) Local Authority Social Services Letter LASSL 4 www.dh.gov. uk, accessed 31/07/06

Gazzard B (2002) *AIDS Care Handbook*, 2nd edn, Mediscript, London

GMC (General Medical Council) (2001) Good Practice Guidelines, Intimate Examinations, www.generalmedicalcouncil.co.uk, accessed 25/02/2006

HPA (Health Protection Agency) (2005) Epidemiological Data-Genital Herpes www.hpa.org.uk, accessed 31/07/2006

Holmes K *et al.* (1999) *Sexually Transmitted Diseases*, 3rd edn. McGraw-Hill, New York

6 Examination of the Anus and Oral Cavity

JENNIFER BROWNE AND MATTHEW GRUNDY-BOWERS

THE EXAMINATION OF THE ANUS

JENNIFER BROWNE

THE ANATOMY AND PHYSIOLOGY OF THE RECTUM AND ANUS

The rectum turns downwards and backwards from the recto-sigmoid junction to follow the curve of the sacrum. It passes out of the peritoneal cavity to end 2 cm in front of and below the tip of the coccyx at its junction with the anal canal. The rectum is totally sheathed in longitudinal muscle fibres. The colorectum is lined with columnar epithelium as far as the dentate line in the middle of the anal canal, where sensitive squamous epithelium, in continuity with that of the perineal skin, takes over. In normal subjects there is a 60–105 degree angle between the rectum and the anal canal. The angle is maintained by the puborectalis muscle, which passes backwards from the pubis around the anorectal junction and back to the pubis, so pulling the anorectal junction forwards (Martini, 2004).

The anorectal junction is not a discrete point, but a region of longitudinal mucosal folds extending superiorly from a zone of mucosa that is paler and flatter. This gives the appearance of a horizontal band with teeth: hence the term 'pectinate line'. The mucosal ridges forming the tooth-like character of the line are termed anal folds or columns. At the pectinate line between the base of the anal columns, the muscosa is redundant, and outpockets to form the anal crypt. The epithelium of the anus, i.e., distal to the pectinate line, is characterised by stratified squamous cells of the non-keratinising type (Martini, 2004).

The anal canal is slightly shorter in women than in men (4.6 cm vs. 3.7 cm). Two cylinders of muscle, the internal anal sphincter, which consists of smooth muscle and is responsible for 80 per cent of the resting tone, and the external anal sphincter, surround it. The external sphincter works in harmony with the puborectalis and levator ani of the pelvic floor (Martini, 2004).

Advanced Clinical Skills for GU Nurses. Edited by Matthew Grundy-Bowers and Jonathan Davies
© 2007 John Wiley & Sons Ltd

EXAMINATION OF THE ANUS

Examination of the anus and rectum should only be carried out on those complaining of anal rectal symptoms, those who have receptive anal sex or receptive oro-anal sex, known as rimming, and those having receptive anal use of sex toys or receptive digital anal penetration. A detailed history is important and will provide clues to the diagnosis. All genital examinations should be carried out with tact and sensitivity, and conducted in a thorough and professional manner. Full explanation of the procedure should be carried out prior to examination, to allay patients' fears and for consent from the patient obtained (Walsh et al., 1999).

An examination should only take place in a private area/room that can be secured to prevent entry to the room during the examination. Good lighting and the use of gloves is essential. Gloves are not only important because of universal precautions but also to re–enforce the clinical nature of the examination (Epstein et al., 2000). All patients should be offered a chaperone when having an intimate examination (Epstein et al., 2000). It is good practice to have a chaperone present for professional and legal reasons. If a patient declines to have a chaperone present this should be documented in the clinical notes. If the clinician feels uncomfortable carrying out an intimate examination without a chaperone, the clinician can refuse to examine the patient.

The patient after explanation of the procedure should be given privacy to undress and a blanket, cover or gown to maintain dignity. Patients should be placed in the left lateral position. With good lighting, firstly inspect the anal skin.

Findings on anal inspection

Pruritus ani, perianal warts, perianal abscess, perianal haematoma, prolapsing haemorrhoids, thrombosed haemorrhoids, skin tags, anal discharge, anal fistulas, anal fissures, anal cancer, rectocele, rectal prolapse, threadworms, faecal soiling of the perineum are all possible findings (Rhodes & Hsin, 1995; Barkauskas, 2002).

The anal tone can be observed at rest and on voluntary contraction. The patient should be asked to strain down as if opening bowels to show perianal descent, prolapsing haemorrhoids or protruding lesions such as tumours or rectal prolapse (Barkauskas, 2002).

Proctoscopy

When preparing the patient for a proctoscope examination, thorough explanation of the examination is needed during the consultation and consent must be obtained. The patient should be placed in the left lateral position, with their knees drawn in to the chest. The proctoscope should be well lubricated with a water-based gel and passed gently into the anus. The patient will feel pressure as the proctoscope comes into contact with the external sphincter; ask the patient to relax and gently pass the proctoscope into the rectum. If there is resistance remove the instrument and allay the patient's fear.

Note on inspection: Faecal matter (if present), odour and consistency. Rectal discharge, threadworms, inflammation, mucosal ulceration, bleeding, haemorrhoids and any other abnormalities. Slowly withdrawing the proctoscope observe the haemorrhoidal cushions, the dentate line, and the anal epithelium.

Patients complaining of rectal bleeding: consider

Blood spotting after anal sex and/or blood spotting on the toilet paper is a common compliant in the GU clinic, and is usually the symptom of minor conditions such as haemorrhoids, anal fissures, genital trauma, or genital warts – which can be associated with pruritus (Rhodes & Hsin, 1995).

Blood separate from faeces is most commonly due to haemorrhoids, but may also be due to a variety of other causes, including rectal carcinoma and proctitis, which can be associated with a mucous discharge. Is the blood fresh – bright red, or old – darkish brown: this can help indicate where the bleeding is from. When does the patient notice it? A proctoscopy should be carried out, but it may be that further investigation may be needed outside of our realm of care, in which case refer appropriately. Blood mixed with faeces may be due to Crohn's disease, or inflammatory bowel disease, carcinoma or vascular abnormalities, and the patient should be referred for careful investigation via a gastroenterologist (Rhodes & Hsin, 1995).

PAIN

Is the pain anal?

This is commonly associated with anal fissures or prolapsed or thrombosed haemorrhoids, which can be easily examined for and diagnosed. Haemorrhoids are usually the result of enlargement of the normal anal cushions. Sometimes undiagnosed herpes lesions, which the patient has not been able to inspect, can be the cause (Hopcroft & Forte, 2003).

Rectal pain

The most commonly complained of rectal pain is intermittent severe rectal pain that is not associated with defecation but may wake the sleeping patient. It is difficult to explain and does not usually result from organic disease. In men prostatitis is a common cause of rectal pain: symptoms include perianal pain. Rectal pain will be worse on defecation (Hopcroft & Forte, 2003).

Pelvic pain

Pelvic pain is a common presentation in women. Pelvic Inflammatory Disease, ectopic pregnancy, endometriosis, ovarian pathology, uterine/cervical cancer and other gynaecological conditions need to be excluded. Often there is no obvious cause found, and often the pain can be a variant of the irritable bowel syndrome (Hopcroft & Forte, 2003).

In the event of no obvious cause, work with the patient to see if there is any underlying cause: are there any pressures relating to sex or any physiological problems, and refer appropriately.

TENESMUS

... is the feeling of incomplete evacuation or a frequent sensation of the need to evacuate. Diarrhoea is often commonly associated, whether it has a functional or an organic cause. These can be signs of rectal disease, including rectal tumours or a large polyp, and can form unpleasant symptoms in ulcerative proctitis (Rhodes & Hsin, 1995).

The rectal ulcer

Syphilis, lympho-granuloma venereum (LGV), or even a solitary herpetic lesion can be the cause (Holmes et al., 1990; Morse et al., 2003). Take appropriate specimens for culture and investigation. The single ulcer causing tenesmus is often related to rectal mucosal prolapse, which would need the intervention of a gastroenterologist or a surgeon (Rhodes & Hsin, 1995).

DISCHARGE

Spontaneous discharge of pus can indicate a sexually transmitted infection or anal or rectal disease. Examination and appropriate specimens should be obtained. Careful inspection should reveal anal tumours, fissuring, and perianal fistula or perianal infections such as perianal warts, syphilitic chancre, and herpetic ulceration (Holmes et al., 1990; Morse et al., 2003).

INCONTINENCE

Incontinence can occur in the presence of a normal sphincter if there is severe diarrhoea. Consultation is needed to assess recent travel abroad, recent diet or change in sexual partner and current sexual practices. The clinician should obtain a stool sample for microscopy and culture. Blood tests for Hepatitis A, B, and C should he undertaken (BASHH, 2005a), but these tests usually do not have an early detection rate, so there should be referral to a senior doctor or an infectious diseases unit if there are other hepatic symptoms and/or hepatitis is suspected. Usually, however, diarrhoea is due to poor sphincter function. Diagnosis depends on an assessment of the three components of sphincter function, the puborectalis sling, the internal and the external sphincter. Incontinence can be related to obstetric trauma, which may have gone unnoticed immediately following the birth.

ANAL LESIONS

Sexually transmitted infections need to be considered in anal lesions/ulceration. Herpetic ulcers/lesions can cause tenesmus and severe pain (BASHH, 2001b; Morse *et al.*, 2003), whereas the syphilitic ulcers/lesions known as chancres are painless in nature (BASHH, 2002b; Holmes *et al.*, 1990). Herpetic lesions/ulcers may look like clusters of blisters or healing sores, but often their appearance can be atypical. With syphilitic lesions in primary syphilis there is often one solitary circular sore; but again this is not always the case. Swabs for *Herpes simplex* virus, microscopy and culture should be obtained, and dark-ground microscopy should be performed on wet mounts of serum and saline for *Treponema pallidum* as well as syphilis serology, which may have to be repeated in early suspected syphilis. Condylomata lata are mucosal lesions in secondary syphilis and tend to have a flatter appearance than anal warts, which are more papilliferous by nature (Holmes *et al.*, 1990; Morse *et al.*, 2003).

Fissured, macular and ulcerating lesions should be biopsied. Paget's and Bowen's diseases can only be diagnosed via histology, and are malignant diseases. Fistulas and perianal abscesses are easy to diagnose on examination. A main problem with this manifestation is not to recognise the possibility of underlying Crohn's disease, especially with the presence of thickened purplish skin tags, and another failing can be to assess the full extent of the fistula inaccurately. Further investigation by a specialist is commonly needed (Rhodes & Hsin, 1995).

The possibility of malignant tumours' being present in the anal canal means that there is a need for the exclusion of carcinomatous diseases: appropriate investigation, referral and management must be carried out.

ANAL WARTS

... are generally sexually transmitted and should alert suspicion to other sexually transmitted infections' being present. Offering a routine sexual health screen to all attending patients complaining of rectal symptoms can exclude these (BASHH, 2002a).

MOLLUSCUM CONTAGIOSUM

Molluscum contagiosum (MC) is caused by a pox virus and typically presents as umbilicated papular lesions: they are quite distinctive, and can be diagnosed on examination. MC is normally sexually transmitted in adults through skin to skin contact (Holmes *et al.*, 1990; BASHH, 2003).

ANAL FISSURES

Patients may complain of severe pain during defecation, sometimes associated with bright red rectal bleeding. Fissures can be easily diagnosed by examination; however, all fissures in men who have sex with men should be screened for LGV, dark ground microscopy on three samples is recommended and syphilis serology.

ANAL TAGS

Anal tags are normal skin variation, and though they do not cause any symptoms or require treatment, sometimes they may be a clue to an underlying condition. As has earlier been stated, tags can be associated with Crohn's disease: these tags are usually thick with a purplish appearance. Anal tags can occur as the result of a thrombosed external pile or may form the marked end to a chronic anal fissure.

PRURITUS

Patients complaining of perianal itching should be further questioned to assess if there are other symptoms such as pain, discharge, rashes or bumps or any sexual contact or family member with similar symptoms. The perianal area and anus should be examined for genital warts, which often cause itching. Is there inflammation in the area? Could there be a candidal infection? Is there similar inflammation and excoriation in other genital areas, the vulva, the penis? With women, is there a thick creamy discharge from the vagina? Appropriate samples should be obtained for analysis.

Phthirus pubis and scabies

Phthirus pubis (pubic lice) and scabies can cause severe itching. Pubic lice can be diagnosed by the presence of lice in the pubic hair. Scabies usually causes an itchy rash all over the body except for the face. The classic sign of burrows can be found on the skin, but primarily between the fingers. Diagnosis of these infestations can be confirmed by microscopy (BASHH, 2001a; Holmes *et al.*, 1990).

Parasites and ova

Parasites such as threadworm are a common cause of pruritus ani in children. Often with adults recent travel is a common factor. Diagnosis is made by observing worms in stool samples or by the sticky-tape test (apply tape to perianal skin and observe under a microscope for eggs). Any suspicion should be confirmed by laboratory testing a stool sample for parasites and ova.

SKIN CONDITIONS

For more detailed information please refer to Chapter 5: The skin and lymphatic system. The skin should be inspected for psoriasis. Is there plaque? Is it bright red rather than mauve or pink. Is it scaly? Look at scalp, fingernails, natal cleft and rest of the skin for any signs of psoriasis; and, importantly, has the patient ever been diagnosed with a skin condition (Seidal *et al.*, 2002).

Eczema

. . . can present with vulval, scrotal, perianal itching with poorly defined itchy pink papules and plaques, with excoriation and scaling. Referral to a specialist genito-urinary consultant or dermatologist will be needed; some clinicians hold joint clinics (Ashton & Leppard, 2005).

Irritant contact dermatitis

. . . can occur as a result of perfumed panty-liners or other chemicals put on the skin. Make a check of changes in washing products, etc. (Ashton & Leppard, 2005).

Allergic contact dermatitis

Often due to applied medicated creams, containing lanolin, for example, antibiotics or contraceptive pessaries/creams, or flavoured lubricants or deodorants. Presentation includes vesicles, weeping and crusting. The skin may be sore rather than itchy. Dermatological referral for management and patch-testing will be required (Ashton & Leppard, 2005).

Lichen sclerosus

Lichen sclerosus is an itchy condition that affects the vulva or the perianal skin. It generally occurs in girls or middle-aged women. In children symptoms are itching, soreness or blisters. It self-resolves in puberty. In older women symptoms are an intolerable itching, soreness and sometimes dypareunia. Classic white atrophic papules and plaques can be seen on the skin; sometimes haemorrhagic blisters and follicular plugging are also present (Ashton & Leppard, 2005).

Finally, poor hygiene can be a cause of anal pruritus; this can be assessed on examination and is easily remedied.

EXAMINATION OF THE ORAL CAVITY

MATTHEW GRUNDY-BOWERS

INTRODUCTION

In most sexual health settings examination of the oral cavity is often forgotten, and when it is made it is often brief. However, examination of the mouth can yield important clinical information, which can be essential in making a diagnosis. It can aid the diagnosis of many conditions from syphilis to HIV and AIDS (Toghill, 1994).

WHEN YOU SHOULD UNDERTAKE AN EXAMINATION

An examination should be undertaken in patients who present with oral symptoms or if it is indicated by the history, as in patients with Lichen planus or syphilis. Patients often present to the clinic with a sore throat following oral sex, concerned that they have contracted a sexually transmitted infection (STI) – especially, for example, if they have performed oral sex for the first time, had sexual contact outside an established relationship or had sexual contact with a sex worker. These symptoms are rarely caused by an STI, and antibiotics are hardly ever indicated. Note that most infections of gonorrhoea are asymptomatic in the throat (BASHH, 2005b), and it is often missed on culture because of poor swabbing technique. It is important to remember that a trivial symptom occasionally heralds a serious problem (Hopcroft & Forte, 2003), and symptoms reported in the mouth should not be taken in isolation, as they may be a feature of generalised disease (Toghill, 1994). Therefore, once an STI is excluded further investigation with a dental practitioner and/or general practitioner may be prudent. Some patients, however, can appear deflated because a sexual cause cannot be found; these patients may need gentle encouragement to seek further medical advice to ensure that a more serious condition is not missed.

THE EXAMINATION

There are four aspects to examination: inspection, palpitation, auscultation and percussion. During the examination of the mouth, oral cavity and throat in sexual health, only inspection and palpation are used (Barkauskas, 2002). During the consultation you may have already picked up on hoarseness and bad breath. Examine the patient sitting down in a chair or on a couch (Swash, 2001), and have a good light source, gloves and a tongue depressor handy. Take a few moments to observe the patient to see if there are any obvious signs such as jaundice, asymmetry or ulceration of the lips (Barkauskas, 2002).

Lymphatic system

Palpate the cervical lymph nodes for evidence of lymphadenopathy, recording the location of nodes and the presence of tenderness. One may find it easier to palpate the cervical lymph nodes by standing behind the patient. For more detailed information about examination of the lymphatic system please refer to Chapter 5.

Inspection of the lips and face

If this is indicated by the history, inspect the eyes for signs of jaundice (BASHH, 2005a), and to see if they are bloodshot or if there is discharge (Barkauskas, 2002). Patients with extensive *Phthirus pubis* (public lice) may occasionally have lice in their eyebrows and eyelashes (BASHH, 2001a). Note if there are any molluscum contagiosum (MC) lesions (BASHH, 2003) on the face or any warts around the mouth (BASHH, 2002a). There is anecdotally evidence that MC facial lesions are associated with HIV, and they can be large and extensive (BASHH, 2003). Then closely examine the lips for:

- Syphilitic primary chancre (BASHH, 2002b)
- Cheilitis (fissuring with scaling and crust formation of the lips), commonly known as chapped lips and caused by sunlight, the cold or wind. This is very common in patients who have had unusual exposure to the elements, such as skiers or fishermen (Swash, 2001; Toghill, 1994).
- Angular stomatitis or cheilosis (cracks in the angles of the mouth) (Swash, 2001): this can be caused by dental appliances such as dentures or braces. It may also be due to malabsorption states (Swash, 2001; Toghill, 1994).
- Impetigo: erythematous base, crusted, yellow, and painless but itching, often accompanied by satellite lesions. Sometimes it is mistaken for herpes, and it is commonly caused by *Staphylococcus aureus* (Prodigy Website, 2002).

Examination of the oral cavity

Ask the patient to open their mouth. Use a good light source and a tongue depressor as a retractor. Systematically inspect the buccal mucosa and between the lower and upper lips and gums (Barkauskas, 2002). If the patient has dentures ask them to remove them. Check for:

- Lichen planus, which presents as *opalescent patches* (Swash, 2001). Check other sites, including the genitals, to confirm.
- Warts.
- Kaposi's sarcoma (Pratt, 2003).

- Oral candidiasis: the lesions are mainly on the soft palate but can extend to the dorsum of the tongue (Toghill, 1994; Walsh *et al.*, 1999). They appear as small white raised points, on an erythematous background (Swash, 2001). It can be seen in patients who have had recent antibiotics or chemotherapy and in those who are immunosuppressed (Walsh *et al.*, 1999).

Ulcers

- Syphilitic primary chancre. This indurated ulcer is normally painless (BASHH, 2002b).
- Snail track ulceration of secondary syphilis (BASHH, 2002b).
- Aphthous ulcers are small superficial painful ulcers with a white or yellow base and a narrow halo of hyperaemia (Swash, 2001). Twenty per cent of the population will suffer with ulcers at some time (Walsh *et al.*, 1999).

Six things to remember about ulcers:

- In elderly patients all mouth ulcers should be considered malignant until proved otherwise (Swash, 2001).
- Mouth ulcers in conjunction with genital ulcers may indicate Behçet's disease (Swash, 2001).
- Don't forget to take a travel history in any patient with an ulcer.
- Any unusual ulcers should be reviewed by a senior medical colleague or referred to a dermatologist for biopsy.
- In high-risk groups an ulcer is syphilis until proved otherwise.
- Ulcers should be palpated to check for induration (Barkauskas, 2002).

Check the tongue for:

- Furring, which is a reasonably common presentation and it is of little clinical significance (Swash, 2001). However, anxious patients often attribute it to HIV infection, concerned that it is either oral *Candida* or oral hairy leukoplakia. This furring is common in smokers (Swash, 2001) and can be caused by patients sleeping with their mouth open, causing their saliva to dry on the tongue. This can easily be removed with a toothbrush.
- Oral hairy leukoplakia: this is normally on the underside of the tongue. It appears as whitish opaque areas of thickened epithelium (Swash, 2001), the patches being of various sizes (Walsh *et al.*, 1999). It is considered pre-malignant (Walsh *et al.*, 1999), and can be an indication of HIV (Pratt, 2003).
- Ulceration.

Finally, inspect the tonsillar bed and oropharynx for erythema, exudates or postnasal discharge. The tonsils and the lymphoid follicles on the back of the oropharynx are often prominent in young subjects. If this is occluded ask the patient to say 'Ah': this will increase visibility (Swash, 2001; Walsh *et al.*, 1999). Unilateral vesicles may indicate *Herpes zoster*. A hole in the hard palate may indicate tertiary syphilis (Swash, 2001). Ulcers on the tonsils may be suggestive of glandular fever, streptococcal tonsillitis, thrombocytopenia, rubella or diphtheria (Swash, 2001). If an abscess is noted it could be quinsy (Swash, 2001; Walsh *et al.*, 1999).

PRESENTATIONS AND COMMON CAUSES

Sore throat

This is probably the most common presentation (Hopcroft & Forte, 2003).

Bad taste and malodorous breath

Possible sources include:

- Poor dental hygiene (Hopcroft & Forte, 2003)
- Smoking (Hopcroft & Forte, 2003)
- Infections of the mouth, such as gingivitis (Toghill, 1994; Hopcroft & Forte, 2003)
- Infections of the mouth and respiratory tract, such as bronchiectasis (Toghill, 1994; Hopcroft & Forte, 2003)
- Medication: the patient may be taking drugs such as metronidazole (Toghill, 1994; Hopcroft & Forte, 2003).

Table 3 Potential causes of sore throats (Hopcroft & Forte, 2003)

Common causes	Occasional causes	Rare causes
• Mild viral pharyngitis • Tonsillitis/streptococcal pharyngitis ('strep throat') • Glandular fever • Quinsy (peritonsillar abcess) • Oropharyngeal candidiasis	• Gastro-oesophageal reflux disease • Glosso-pharyngeal neuralgia and cervicogenic nerve root pain • Trauma (foreign body or scratch from badly chewed crispy food) • Other viral or bacterial infections, e.g. Vincent's angina, herpangina, *Herpes simple*, gonorrhoea • Aphthous ulceration • Acute or sub-acute thyroiditis	• Cardiac angina • Carotodynia • Blood dyscrasia (including iatrogenic) • Epiglottitis • Diphtheria • Oro-pharyngeal carcinoma • Retro-pharyngeal abscess

Soreness of the tongue

Possible sources include:

- Trauma (Hopcroft & Forte, 2003)
- Anaemia (Hopcroft & Forte, 2003)
- Pernicious anaemia and mucositis due to chemotherapy (Toghill, 1994)
- Idiopathic (? mechanical) soreness (Toghill, 1994).

SUMMARY

Examination of the mouth can be extremely useful in aiding a diagnosis; however, it is often overlooked. It is important to remember, though, that symptoms can often be a sign of something non-sexual, so referral back to the patient's general practitioner or to a dentist is prudent.

REFERENCES

Ashton R, Leppard B (2005) *Differential Diagnosis in Dermatology*, 3rd edn. Radcliffe Medical Press, Oxford

Barkauskas VH, Baumann LC, Darling Fisher CS (2002) *Health and Physical Assessment.* Mosby, St Louis

BASHH (British Association for Sexual Health and HIV) (2001a) National Guideline for the Management of *Phthirus pubis* Infestations http://www.bashh.org/guidelines/2002/pubic_lice_0901b.pdf **(Accessed 27/02/2006)**

BASHH (British Association for Sexual Health and HIV) (2001b) National Guideline for the Management of Genital Herpes http://www.bashh.org/guidelines/2002/hsv_0601.pdf **(Accessed 27/02/2006)**

BASHH (British Association for Sexual Health and HIV) (2002a) National Guideline for the Management of Anogenital Warts http://www.bashh.org/guidelines/2002/hpv_0302b.pdf **(Accessed 27/02/2006)**

BASHH (British Association for Sexual Health and HIV) (2002b) National Guideline for the Management of Early Syphilis http://www.bashh.org/guidelines/2002/early$final0502.pdf **(Accessed 27/02/2006)**

BASHH (British Association for Sexual Health and HIV) (2003) National Guideline for the Management of Molluscum Contagiosum http://www.bashh.org/guidelines/2002/c12_0403c.pdf **(Accessed 27/02/2006)**

BASHH (British Association for Sexual Health and HIV) (2005a) National Guideline for the Management of Viral Hepatitides A, B & C http://www.bashh.org/guidelines/2005/hepatitis_abc_final_0905.pdf **(Accessed 27/02/2006)**

BASHH (British Association for Sexual Health and HIV) (2005b) National Guideline for the Diagnosis and Treatment of Gonorrhoea in Adults http://www.bashh.org/guidelines/2005/gc_final_0805.pdf **(Accessed 27/02/2006)**

Epstein O, Perkin DG, de Bono DP, Cookson J (2000) *Clinical Examination*, 2nd edn. Mosby, St Louis

Holmes KK et al. (1990) *Sexually Transmitted Diseases*, 2nd edn. McGraw Hill, New York

Hopcroft K, Forte V (2003) *Symptom Sorter*, 2nd edn. Radcliffe Medical Press, Oxford

Martini FH (2004) *Fundamentals of Anatomy and Physiology*, 6th edn. Benjamin Cummings, San Francisco

Morse SA *et al.* (2003) *Altas of Sexually Transmitted Diseases and AIDS*, 3rd edn. Mosby, London

Pratt R (2003) *AIDS: A Strategy for Nursing Care*, 5th edn. Edward Arnold, London

Prodigy Website (2002) Impetigo Quick Reference Guide http://www.prodigy.nhs.uk/ProdigyKnowledge/QRG/Content/pdfs/QR%20Impetigo.pdf **(Accessed 27/02/2006)**

Rhodes JM, Hsin Tsai H (1995) *Clinical Problems in Gastroenterology*, Mosby-Wolfe, London

Seidal HM, Ball JW, Dains JE, Benedict GW (2002) *Mosby's Guide to Physical Examination*. Mosby, St Louis

Swash M (2001) *Hutchinson's Clinical Methods*. WB Saunders, Edinburgh

Toghill P (1994) *Examining patients: an introduction to clinical medicine*. Edward Arnold, London

Walsh M, Crumbie A, Reveley S (1999) *Nurse Practitioners: Clinical Skills and Professional Issues*. Butterworth Heinemann, Oxford

7 Legal Issues in Sexual Health

JONATHAN DAVIES

INTRODUCTION

Since its launch in 1948 the National Health Service has been an organisation that has continuously evolved and grown. It has developed in response to political, economic and social factors and in addition the added pressures of medical advancement. The changes can be seen in every element of the services provided, from increasing evidence-based practice through to a transparent and open delivery of care. At this time more than ever healthcare professionals will be working to deliver health care within this dynamic environment, and thereby carry a responsibility to protect the public and to provide health care that is both current and up-to-date.

Even though the provision of health care has changed and expanded over the past fifty years, the core principle of free access to health care remains solid. It is clear within this ever-developing service that major areas that need to respond to changes are the professional roles. Arguably no single profession has changed and expanded so considerably as the role of the Nurse.

This can be seen in a role as commonplace as the Nurse Practitioner: once considered unique and specialist, it is slowly becoming a feature of, and established within, sexual health clinics throughout the UK. Many services now depend on the nurse to deliver specialist care in an autonomous and professional manner. Increasing demands on services fuelled by a continuing rise in STIs drive the demand for care and in turn for more creative ways of practice.

As a response to the rise in sexually transmitted infections the government in the UK has explored and considered the Sexual Health of the nation and as a result formulated new policy and guidelines that will further shape nursing practice. The sexual health strategy (DH 2001a) and more recently the 'choosing health' document, published in November 2004 (DH 2004a) place sexual health as a core element in the health of our society. Amongst their aims is 48-hour access to a sexual heath clinic (DH 2004a), a target that in some parts of the country cannot be met with the present availability of services. Additionally there is also the roll out of the National *Chlamydia* Screening Programming (DH 2004b), designed to capture the young people who are

Advanced Clinical Skills for GU Nurses. Edited by Matthew Grundy-Bowers and Jonathan Davies
© 2007 John Wiley & Sons Ltd

statistically the most at risk of contracting this commonly silent infection (Health Protection Agency 2005). More recently community pharmacies are being encouraged to become involved and test young people (DH 2005).

It is becoming clear, then, that sexual health nursing delivered within the framework of the NHS is part of the changing and dynamic system that affects other forms of health care. The increasing pool of sexually transmitted infections drives demands for services that are presently under review and being updated. It is with this in mind that nursing will continue to meet the challenge. At the forefront of new roles and working practices the nursing profession must continue with a responsive and professional approach to sexual health. It is important therefore to look at the new roles and consider the professional and legal responsibilities that encapsulate them. The eagerness and enthusiasm that is demonstrated by the nursing profession must continue to move forwards, and in harmony with this the profession must consider its position legally and professionally and continue to protect the public and enhance the reputation and role of the specialist sexual health nurse within today's NHS.

It is important to recognise the wide range of legal and professional issues that influence nursing practice. For the purpose of this chapter the focus will be on the common issues that affect sexual health nursing practice. These legal and professional issues are both vast and varied. The chapter aims to address the most relevant and challenging issues that sexual health nurses encounter in their daily practice.

• Confidentiality
• Consent to treatment
• Treatment of young people

It is important to acknowledge that the scope of the chapter does not allow for a full and varied explanation of all the legal and professional issues faced in sexual health, and also that the law and its application can evolve and change each time a new legal challenge is raised. It is therefore essential to consider this chapter in terms of an exploration of the legal issues faced in practice and not as a guide on the basis of which concrete decisions regarding practice are made. The chapter should be used to generate thoughts and discussion in consideration of practice.

CONFIDENTIALITY

More than any other area of health care the delivery of sexual health nursing is bound by the broad principles of patient confidentiality. The need for public trust is a foundation of any nurse–patient relationship. To elicit a deeply personal sexual history without complete confidence would be a difficult and stressful task. In a wider context the need for confidentiality is implicit, and without the trust and confidence of the public few people would come forward for testing within sexual health clinics for fear of being identified.

Sexual health or genito-urinary medicine clinics, as they are also known, are bound by legislation that ensures confidentiality and governs the operation of the clinic. The National Health Service Act (1977) provides a legal framework that imposes upon the Secretary of State a number of obligations to provide free health care. As with accident and emergency services, treatment for sexually transmitted infections is free in the United Kingdom. All consultations are treated in the strictest confidence, and patients may use a pseudonym or give no name at all.

The Venereal Disease Regulations (1974) 'place a duty on health authorities to ensure that any information capable of identifying an individual examined or treated for any sexually transmitted disease shall not be disclosed'. The 1974 regulation has now been updated under The NHS Trusts and Primary Care Trusts (Sexually Transmitted Diseases) Directions (2000). Sexual health clinics are quite unique in having this specific legislation put in place to maintain the confidentiality of those attending for treatment. There is no other specific NHS service that has this provision in addition to the normal frameworks for maintaining patient confidentiality.

DEFINITIONS OF CONFIDENTIALITY

When using the law, and specifically case law, to test and challenge notions it is common to use examples that although at first seem far removed from health care have the same core principles in their argument. It is important to ascertain what information is confidential and what constitutes a breach thereof. In the case of *Marshall v Guinle Ltd (1979)*, an industrial case that examined employees using confidential business information to set themselves up in competition, a definition of confidential information was provided:

'The information must be of such a nature that its release would be injurious to the owner or of advantage to others.
The owner must believe the information is confidential or secret.
The owner's belief under these headings must be reasonable.
The information must be judged in the light of usages and practices in the particular industry concerned' (cited in Kennedy & Grubb 2000).

It would therefore be reasonable to argue that similar principles could be applied to the belief of patients with reference to information held about them. Also it should be safe to assume that the healthcare worker is aware that the information is of a confidential nature and that to pass such information on would be a breach of such confidentiality.

In England and Wales there is generally a common law duty of confidentiality imposed upon doctors and nurses, the reasons for which are manifold. The obligation for confidentiality was discussed in *A-G v Guardian Newspa-*

pers Ltd (No. 2) (1988). This judgement 'affirmed that there was a public interest in a legally enforceable protection of confidences received under notice of confidentiality' (Mason & McCall Smith 1999). In this case the judge, Lord Goff, summarised the law in the following way:

> I start with the broad general principle. . . . That a duty of confidence arises when confidential information comes to the knowledge of a person (the confidant) in circumstances where he has notice, or is held to have agreed, that the information is confidential, with the effect that it would be just in all the circumstances that he should be precluded from disclosing the information to others (*A-G v Guardian Newspapers Ltd (No. 2) 1988).*

This statement appears quite clear; and if executed in the business setting where sensitive commercial information is passed around and contracts exchanged it is indeed reasonably straightforward. However, in the context of the doctor–patient relationship in the NHS there is no such contractual relationship existing between the two parties Kennedy and Grubb (2000, p. 1060).

SO HOW THEN DOES THE COMMON LAW OF CONFIDENTIALITY GOVERN HEALTHCARE WORKERS?

It is a basic responsibility of medical and nursing practice that the confidentiality of all patients is maintained in the course of one's duty and as stipulated in Mason and McCall Smith (1999, p. 191): 'A general common law duty is imposed on a doctor to respect the confidences of his patients.' This would therefore suggest that the responsibility of the duty of confidentiality is rigid, and that there is no option other than to maintain it no matter what the circumstances.

BREACHING CONFIDENTIALITY

Having considered the duty of confidentiality and its importance and rigidity, when may there be a circumstance when the need for confidentiality can be challenged? Perhaps in a climate where knowingly passing on the HIV virus has become a criminal act (*R v Adaye (2004), R v Dica (2003), R v Konzani (2004)),* this absolute view of the confidential nurse–patient relationship must be brought into question. As a nurse engaging patients in the process of testing for HIV, what should one do when the scenario arises where you, the healthcare professional, are fully aware of a client's HIV diagnosis and also have the knowledge that they are having unprotected sex with their regular partner. To some, this scenario may sound extreme and far-fetched; yet to many who work in sexual health clinics it is a situation that seems to arise with greater and greater frequency. The recent emergence of successful prosecutions for knowingly passing on the HIV virus is considered a worrying trend in some quarters. Perhaps the same legal principles could be applied to other Sexually

Transmitted Infections, thus opening up the floodgates for multiple court cases, and as a result damaging the reputation of the sexual health services.

UNDER WHAT CIRCUMSTANCES CAN CONFIDENTIALITY BE BREACHED OR CHALLENGED?

Having given consideration to the broad principles that protect confidentiality in the clinical setting, it is relevant also to explore circumstances in which the normal boundaries of patient confidentiality may be encroached upon or challenged. Let's consider what are probably the only two straightforward situations where a healthcare professional may justify passing on confidential information. The first may be when the patient gives their consent to do so, and the second when it is in the public interest to do so.

Let's examine this further

There is an exception in the venereal disease regulations: this allows doctors to share information regarding their patients with other clinics. The regulation states that all information must remain confidential except 'for the purpose of communicating that information to a medical practitioner, or to a person employed under the direction of a medical practitioner in connection with the treatment of persons suffering from such disease or the prevention of the spread thereof, and for the purpose of such treatment or prevention' (National Health Service Act 1977). It must be acknowledged that the aim of such legislation is to protect the confidentiality of individuals and therefore encourage them to attend. The exception, however, allows doctors or nurses and Health Advisers employed under their guidance to explore the concept of partner notification for the individual with an STI. Is it possible then to breach their confidentiality in order to prevent the further spread of disease?

In the context of the recent cases where individuals have been found guilty of knowingly passing on the HIV virus, let us explore the legal and professional issues that may arise for the practitioner. First, let's examine the potential duty of the healthcare worker who is aware of the HIV status of their patient. What obstacles stand in their way in breaching confidentiality, and what, if any, may be the advantages? Taking recent professional experience into account, there have been examples of situations where this would seem to be the right thing to do in order to protect a sexual partner from these diseases.

Arguments against breaching confidentiality

There are of course a number of factors that would prohibit the healthcare worker from informing a patient's partner, the vital one being that of patient confidentiality. Both the medical and nursing professions have codes of professional conduct that prohibit them from disclosing details of patients' treatment and consultations with others. The Hippocratic Oath states: 'All that may come to my knowledge in the exercise of my profession or outside my profession or in daily commerce with men that ought not to be spread abroad, I will keep secret and will never reveal' (cited in Mason *et al.* 2002, p. 243), and the General Medical Council offers more recent guidance: 'Patients have a right to expect that information about them will be held in confidence by their doctors. Confidentiality is central to trust between doctors and patients. Without assurances about confidentiality, patients may be reluctant to give doctors the information they need in order to provide good care' (GMC 1998). Equally, the nursing profession are bound by their professional code of conduct: 'You must treat information about patients and clients as confidential and use it only for the purpose for which it was given' (Nursing and Midwifery Council 2004). The codes of conduct and their similar themes interweave confidentiality into everything that doctors and nurses do.

The common argument to support this is that without a strict guarantee of confidentiality patients may disclose less about themselves and their conditions, as a result of which the treatment that they receive may be inferior to that which is required. To consider this in the field of sexual health, confidentiality and the practitioner–patient relationship is of crucial importance. A typical consultation with a sexual health doctor or nurse will call for disclosure of a number of intimate details that include: sexual orientation, details of sexual partners, types of sexual practices, previously diagnosed sexually transmitted infections (STIs), and whether or not safer sex practices were used.

It is important to acknowledge that being armed with this sensitive information regarding a patient's sexual history may put the individual into a very vulnerable position. Therefore a strong ethos of confidentiality within the therapeutic relationship is required. If, as in the legal case of *R v Kelly (2001)*, the police obtain a warrant to look at the individual's medical history, then firm evidence may be gained to build a case following the transmission of HIV, thereby voiding our promise of confidentiality to our patients and harming our reputation as a service.

So if it were to be the healthcare professional's duty to inform the index patients' partner of the HIV diagnosis, how would they overcome the obvious hurdle posed by their professional obligation to respect patient confidentiality? In addition to this, HIV services under the umbrella of sexual health clinics lead patients to believe that all information given remains confidential. The author would argue that patients would confidently assume that they would be treated in the strictest confidence on engaging with the service, holding the belief that the information is confidential or secret (*Marshall (Thomas) (Exports) Ltd v Guinle 1979*).

It would be easy for the patient to assume that in England a right to privacy may exist in statute or as a result of the evolution of case law. Until recently it has been considered that 'there is no right to privacy in English law, although in practice much that is private can be protected in other ways' (Staunch & Wheat 1998, p. 225). Therefore people can gain legal remedy for such a breach, using, for example, the tort of trespass. In 1998 the European Convention on Human Rights (1998) became part of English law. Article 8 of the Act offers protection for a right to private life. The use of these legal remedies may also imply to the patient that 'Confidential' means confidential. If healthcare workers were to take the lead in breaching that right, then on what grounds could they proceed?

When could it be justified that one shares confidential patient information?

Although the patient often assumes confidentiality, there do appear to be contradictions in its application. Obviously with the relevant patient's expressed consent a doctor can safely share confidential information in appropriate circumstances. There are specific professional guidelines laid down by the GMC as to when it is right to disclose information concerning individuals and their care. Included in the document is the guidance on disclosing information in the public interest: 'in cases where patients withhold consent, personal information may be disclosed in the public interest where the benefits to an individual or to society of the disclosure outweigh the patient's interest in keeping the information confidential' (GMC 2004). The guidelines therefore suggest that doctors can, when it is proved necessary, breach the duty of confidentiality to their patient.

Examples of breaching confidentiality can be seen in other case law concerning breaches of confidence, and may be useful when drawing comparisons. In the case of *W v Egdell (1990)* cited in Staunch and Wheat (1998, p. 239) a secure hospital prisoner made an application for transfer to a regional unit; this was considered to be a step towards discharge. His legal team sought the opinion of a psychiatrist to support the application. In the opinion of Dr Egdell the patient was considered dangerous, and as a result his application was withdrawn. Soon after, his case was up for an automatic review under s79 of the Mental Health Act 1983. Dr Egdell, on realising that his report was commissioned by the legal team but might not be included in the patient's medical notes, forwarded his report to the Home Office and the hospital's medical director.

The patient in question brought a case against Dr Egdell alleging breach of confidence. The court upheld the breach of confidence on the grounds of protecting the public interest, and the patient failed in the first instance and subsequently appealed. The court of appeal 'unanimously confirmed the trial judge's decision to dismiss the action but did so with rather more reservation' (Mason *et al.* 2002, p. 246). Further consideration was such that patients such as 'W' should enjoy the same confidence as other members of the public in order to 'bare his soul and open his mind', and that anything less would be 'contrary to the public interest'.

On consideration of the case the author would argue that Dr Egdell clearly breached the concept of confidentiality between himself and 'W'. This breach of confidentiality is clearly a paternalistic practice on the part of the medical practitioner. This is given as an extreme example of a situation where the need to protect the public directly overrides the right to confidentiality of the individual. The court of appeal rightly expressed concern as to the rights of 'W', and balanced them against the greater good and the public interest. It should be only with great caution that practitioners actively breach confidentiality, because, once information regarding a patient is made public, the damage to the individual is done, and is often irreversible. What has been told cannot be untold or retracted.

There appear to be times when it is important that we reinforce to patients the confidential nature of our services in order to provide a safe service and improve the health of individuals and the public at large. However, on exploration it becomes apparent that the confidentiality promised isn't always guaranteed. In the light of the growing number of individuals being found guilty of knowingly passing on HIV, professionals in sexual health are faced with the dilemma: how confidential is our promise of confidentiality?

The arguments to maintain patient confidentiality are strong and robust, and any practitioner faced with a situation in which they feel a strong argument to breach confidentiality should proceed with caution. Wide discussion within the service and advice from relevant legal departments or professional bodies is required to support any decisions to proceed.

ISSUES OF CONSENT

As a practitioner in the sexual health setting it is essential to consider the boundaries and issues of consent to medical treatment. After all, we are engaging clients into a situation where arguably they may feel vulnerable and coerced into agreeing to procedures and tests that they are uncomfortable and unfamiliar with. The expanded role of the nurse places practitioners at the forefront of patient care as never before. The nurse who runs her own sexual health clinic or performs minor operations must familiarise herself with the concepts of consent to treatment in order to practise in a way that is respectful and supportive of the patient as an individual.

Nurses working within the arena of sexual health must give careful consideration to the following judgement. It implies that to perform any kind of procedure without the patient being fully aware of the implications and subsequently offering their total consent would leave the practitioner vulnerable to accusations of assault: 'Every human being of adult years and sound mind has a right to determine what shall be done with his own body; and a surgeon who performs an operation without his patient's consent commits an assault, for which he is liable in damages' (Justice Cardozo cited in Kennedy and Grubb 2000, p. 575).

'The right of a person to control his or her own body is a concept that has long been recognised at common law. The tort of battery has traditionally protected the interest in bodily security from unwanted physical interference. Basically, any intentional non-consensual touching which is harmful or offensive to a person's reasonable sense of dignity is actionable' (Malette v Shuman 1990). The meaning of this judgement appears quite clear, in that without consent any form of interaction with a patient may leave the practitioner vulnerable to legal action.

It becomes clear, then, that consent is a major issue in health care, and for the purpose of this chapter and in the context of sexual health nursing we will examine it in relation to the following:

- Consent to treatment
- Consent from younger people
- Consent to sexual relationships.

CONSENT TO TREATMENT

In order to begin exploring issues of consent let us start by examining a number of definitions. A basic definition of consent follows: 'Voluntary agreement to or acquiescence in what another proposes or desires; compliance, concurrence, permission' (*Shorter Oxford Dictionary*, 3rd edn, 1944). Perhaps this definition suggests that one party should voluntarily agree to, and be familiar with, what another party proposes to do with or for them. The Department of Health states the importance of consent within the context of the NHS: 'Patients have a fundamental legal and ethical right to determine what happens to their own bodies. Valid consent to treatment is therefore absolutely central in all forms of health care, from providing personal care to undertaking major surgery. Seeking consent is also a matter of common courtesy between health professionals and patients' (DH 2001a). Here the Department of Health builds on other definitions and states that the individual has a right to be treated according to the common principle that lies behind them throughout their treatment. In order to clear up the many issues and conflicting standards of consent in the National Health Service the DH issued a document that offered national guidelines on standards in consent. The formulations produced look at the issue from the following perspectives:

- Consenting adults
- Consenting children and young people
- Consenting people with learning disabilities
- Consent, a guide for parents.

All of these documents are available from the Department of Health at their website. The main document, entitled *Reference Guide to Consent for Examination or Treatment* (DH 2001b), also sets out guidelines for practitioners when engaging patients in research trials or medical photography and, importantly in the field of sexual health, when soliciting their consent to blood tests.

For the practitioner in sexual health as much as in any other field there are a number of key issues to consider when obtaining the consent of a patient to treatment. Primarily, the patient must be able to give consent, be of an appropriate age and have the mental capacity to do so. It is worth always considering that no adult has the right to consent for another adult who has the capacity to consent for him- or herself. In practice, one of the challenges may be where an individual, perhaps a husband, is translating for another, maybe for his wife. The practitioner involved in this situation would need to be very sure that the patient fully understands what she is consenting to, and in most circumstances it would be more appropriate to have an independent interpreter present.

FORMS OF CONSENT

Express consent is given when the clients clearly state that they wish to undergo a given procedure that the doctor or nurse has fully explained to them. 'Consent is express when the patient explicitly agrees to what is proposed by the doctor. It need not be set out in any specific form and it need not be in writing' (Kennedy & Grubb 2000, p. 583). The DH guidance for consent provides a number of consent forms for a variety of situations. However, written consent is not a requirement of a consent procedure, but it is proof or evidence that the course of treatment was agreed on.

There may be other situations where the patient puts himself or herself forward for treatment where the intricacies of consent have not been discussed: this may be termed **implied consent**. 'On one view, it is said that the law implies consent from the patient's conduct, i.e. deduces his state of mind. Another view which we think more tenable would describe implied consent as something of a fiction' (Kennedy & Grubb 2000, p. 589). Professor John Flemming, cited in Kennedy and Grubb (2000, p. 589), offers the following examples of what may be defined as implied consent: 'Consent may be given expressly, as when a patient authorizes a surgeon to perform an operation, but it may just as well be implied: Actions often speak louder than words. Holding up one's bare arm to a doctor at a vaccination point is as clear an assent as if it were expressed in words.' So here the practitioner can consider the varying degrees and definitions of what actually constitutes consent. Perhaps it would be wise when preparing her practice that the practitioner consider the implications of each procedure that she carries out. Would it be sensible to have written consent for patients who undergo cryotherapy, because of the risk of scarring? Or should we just accept the implied consent of the patient removing their clothing and positioning themselves comfortably to accept treatment?

Alternatively, owing to the life-changing potential of a positive HIV test, should the practitioner obtain written consent, to demonstrate that a dialogue surrounding the issues has taken place? These are questions that the individual practitioner or the clinic in which they work must answer for him-, her-, or itself. It would be wise to prepare any policy by first engaging with the DH materials on consent, which are readily available.

YOUNG PEOPLE

Perhaps one of the most controversial areas of consent for sexual health practitioners is that of young people consenting to examination and treatment. The tests of Gillick competence or Fraser guidelines have for many years been used as the benchmark for young people making autonomous decisions regarding their health. In practice, if a young person is considered competent, then the practitioner can go ahead and provide the treatment that they request. Lord Scarman, cited in Mason *et al.* (2002, p. 319) offers the following affirmation: 'It can be taken as being now accepted that a doctor treating a child should always attempt to obtain parental authority but that, provided the patient is capable of understanding what is proposed and of expressing his or her wishes, the doctor may, in exceptional circumstances, provide treatment on the basis of the minor's consent alone. The decision to do so must be taken on clinical grounds and, clearly, must depend heavily on the severity and permanence of the proposed therapy' (Mason *et al.* 2002, p. 319). Perhaps the 'exceptional circumstances' in the field of sexual health would consist in the need to protect the confidentiality of the individual and their future sexual health. Scarmans final sentence talks of the severity of the therapy, and, as we've seen in recent times, decisions to obtain the consent of minors for terminations of pregnancy have been challenged by their parents in the UK courts.

In order to give further clarity to practitioners the Department of Health released guidelines in 2004 for the treatment of young people: 'Best Practice Guidance For Doctors and other Health Professionals on the Provision of Advice and Treatment to Young People Under 16 on Contraception, Sexual and Reproductive Health' (DH 2004c).

The document clearly sets out the parameters in which the practitioner should work when offering sexual health services to under-sixteens:

> Doctors and health professionals have a duty of care and a duty of confidentiality to all patients, including under 16s. This guidance applies to the provision of advice and treatment on contraception, sexual and reproductive health, including abortion (DH 2004c).

It is considered good practice for doctors and other health professionals to follow the criteria outlined by Lord Fraser in 1985, in the House of Lords' ruling in the case of Victoria Gillick v West Norfolk and Wisbech Health Authority and Department of Health and Social Security. These are commonly known as the Fraser Guidelines: see Box Five.

So here we have some clear guidelines that may support practitioners in their decisions to treat young persons of less than sixteen years of age.

A further dilemma that faces nurses in the area of sexual health is that of young people under sixteen accessing and using sexual health services. The law clearly states that the age of consent for a young person to engage in sexual activity is sixteen; this applies whether they are gay, straight or bisexual. Here then is our first dilemma: if we are offering young people sexual health screenings, distributing condoms and referring them for termination of pregnancy, are we encouraging illegal activity and in danger of coming into conflict with the law? The Sexual Offences Act 2003 (Home Office 2004) does offer some guidance to support practitioners in their work with young people: 'Although the age of consent remains at 16, the law is not intended to prosecute mutually agreed teenage sexual activity between two young people of a similar age, unless it involves abuse or exploitation' (The Sexual Offences Act 2003). The act itself also clears up an area that could become a minefield for sexual health practitioners dealing with young people. The act contains extensive legislation for the purpose of protecting young people. Among this legislation is Section 14 which is headed: 'Arranging or facilitating commission of a child sex offence'; here it is made quite clear that a nurse, doctor or practitioner engaged in treating, protecting or advising a young person in a sexual health service context need not fear being accused of preparing a child for, or assisting a child to commit, a sexual offence. The legislation states that:

Box Five

Prerequisites for the legal provision of contraceptive advice and treatment to young people

- *the young person understands the health professional's advice;*
- *the health professional cannot persuade the young person to inform his or her parents or allow the doctor to inform the parents that he or she is seeking contraceptive advice;*
- *the young person is very likely to begin or continue having intercourse with or without contraceptive treatment;*
- *unless he or she receives contraceptive advice or treatment, the young person's physical or mental health or both are likely to suffer; and*
- *the young person's best interests require the health professional to give contraceptive advice, treatment or both without parental consent.*

Department of Health (2004c)

For the purposes of subsection (2), a person acts for the protection of a child if he acts for the purpose of

(a) protecting the child from sexually transmitted infection,
(b) protecting the physical safety of the child,
(c) preventing the child from becoming pregnant, or
(d) promoting the child's emotional well-being by the giving of advice,

and not for the purpose of obtaining sexual gratification or for the purpose of causing or encouraging the activity constituting the offence within subsection (1)(b) or the child's participation in it (The Sexual Offences Act 2003).

So the inclusion of this specific clause does give the practitioner the confidence to encourage sexually active young people to engage with, and participate in, sexual health services to gain advice and maintain their health.

The Sexual Offences Act contains many areas of sex-related law that are valuable to professionals working within the sexual health fields. Clarification is given on many areas, from rape and assault through to cottaging, voyeurism and indecent exposure. The limitations of this chapter do not allow a full exploration of the Act; however, it is advisable for practitioners to obtain a copy and familiarise themselves with all of its many aspects.

Again the area of consent and its various applications provide a number of challenges to the sexual health practitioner, the most challenging being that of working with young people. Again it is important to use the chapter to stimulate questions and discussions; and when faced with an unclear situation regarding young people you should always seek guidance from others within your team. Ultimately it is essential to remember that the welfare of the child is always paramount.

CONCLUSION

The law in its relationship with sexual health nursing can at times make a confusing and frustrating bedfellow. There is often no right or wrong answer, no guidelines that are set in stone and no easy solution to the many dilemmas and challenges that face nurses within the sexual health setting. This chapter has explored the most common issues that arise in practice: consent and confidentiality. It is of course important to realise that there are many other aspects of law that influence the delivery of care.

As a practitioner in sexual health, facing up to the dilemmas and challenges of practice is something that one can only do satisfactorily when armed with a basic knowledge of legal, and in addition, ethical theory. There are many key texts specifically written for law and health care that will help one to develop and build a working legal knowledge base. It would be dangerous, however, to conclude that, merely by using the basic theories discussed here and in other key texts one could safely proceed to take autonomous decisions that involve legal matters in isolation. It is good practice to seek support from colleagues, management and, in the more complex issues, the national health legal support services.

The multitude of health-related cases that make the newspapers and television can be used and examined when we consider the future delivery of health care. At the time of writing this chapter there are a number of people now convicted of knowingly transmitting HIV, including the first woman to be convicted. As we shall see over the coming months and years, the development of case law will result in pressures to change and shape nursing practice, responding to the issues that arise for consenting clients and promising them confidentiality. As nurses in the provision of an ever-changing healthcare system, it will be important for us to acknowledge and overcome the many challenges and issues that come our way.

REFERENCES

DH (Department of Health) (2001a) *Better Prevention, Better Services, Better Sexual Health – The National Strategy for Sexual Health and HIV Sexual Health Strategy.* DH, London

DH (Department of Health) (2001b) 'Reference Guide to Consent for Examination or Treatment www.dh.gov.uk/PublicationAndstatistics/Publications/ PublicationsPolicyandGuidance/PublicationsPolicyandGuidanceArticle/fs/en? CONTENT_ID=4006757&chk=snmdw8

DH (Department of Health) (2004a) *Choosing Health: Making Healthier Choices Easier*, November. DH, London

DH (Department of Health) (2004b) *The National Chlamydia Screening Programme in England. Programme Overview, Core Requirements and Data Collection*, 2nd edn, April. DH, London

DH (Department of Health) (2004c) *Best Practice Guidance for Doctors and Other Health Professionals on the Provision of Advice and Treatment to Young People under 16 on Contraception, Sexual and Reproductive Health*, July. DH, London

DH (Department of Health) (2005) *Chlamydia Screening on the High Street*, February. DH, London

GMC (General Medical Council) (1998) 'Guidance on Good Practice, Confidentiality', www.gmc-uk.org/ standards/default.htm (accessed 31/08/05)

Home Office (2004) *Children and Families: Safer from Sexual Crime*, May. Home Office Communications Directorate, London

HPA (Health Protection Agency) (2005) *Sexually Transmitted Infections, Epidemiological Data.* Available from: http://www.hpa.org.uk/infections/topics_az/hiv_and_sti/ epidemiology/sti_data/htm (accessed 7/11/2005)

Kennedy I, Grubb A (2000) *Medical Law*, 3rd edn. Butterworth, London

Mason JK, McCall Smith RA (1999) *Law and Medical Ethics*, 5th edn. Butterworth, London

Mason JK, McCall Smith RA, Laurie GT (2002) *Law and Medical Ethics*, 6th edn. Butterworth, London

Nursing and Midwifery Council (2004) 'Code of Professional Conduct: standards of conduct, performance and ethics.' http://www.nmc-uk.org (accessed 31/08/05)
Staunch M, Wheat K (1998) *Sourcebook on Medical Law*. Cavendish Publishing Ltd, London

TABLE OF STATUTES

Human Rights Act 1998
Mental Health Act 1983
National Health Service Act 1977
National Health Service Act 1977, The NHS Trusts and Primary Care Trusts (Sexually Transmitted Diseases) Directions 2000
The Public Health (Infectious Diseases) Regulations 1988
The Sexual Offences Act 2003
The Venereal Disease Regulations (1974)

TABLE OF CASES

A-G v Guardian Newspapers Ltd (No. 2) (1990)
Gillick v West Norfolk and Wisbech Health Authority (1984)
Malette v Shuman (1990) 67 DLR (4th) 321 (Ont CA)
Marshall (Thomas) (Exports) Ltd v Guinle (1979)
R v Adaye (2004)
R v Dica (2003)
R v Kelly (2001)
R v Konzani (2004)
W v Egdell (1990)

WEBSITES

www.aidsmap.com
www.dh.gov.uk
www.gmc-uk.org
www.homeoffice.gov.uk
www.hpa.org
www.lawtel.co.uk
www.lexisnexis.com
www.nhs.uk
www.nmc-uk.org
www.westlaw.co.uk

8 HIV Pre- and Post-Test Discussion

JANE HOOKER

INTRODUCTION

HIV continues to be one of the most important communicable diseases in the UK. It is an infection associated with significant morbidity and mortality, high costs of treatment and care, and high numbers of potential years of life lost. Each year, many thousands of individuals are diagnosed with HIV for the first time.

BRIEF HISTORY OF HIV

When HIV/AIDS was first discovered it was known by many names. By 1982 some people, linking the condition to its initial known occurrence in gay men, called the disease variously 'gay compromise syndrome', 'GRID' *(gay-related immune deficiency)* and 'gay cancer'. The disease was also called *'community-acquired immune dysfunction'*, 'LAV' *(lymphadenopathy-associated virus), and* 'HTLV-3' *(human T-cell lymphotropic virus, type 3)*.

In May 1986, however, the International Committee on the Taxonomy of Viruses ruled that a new name of HIV (Human Immunodeficiency Virus) would be given to this disease.

In December 1981 the first case of AIDS was diagnosed in the UK. By October 1985, UK blood transfusion centres began routine HIV testing of all blood donations (Pratt, 2003).

THE HISTORY OF HIV PRE- AND POST-TEST DISCUSSIONS IN THE UK

Since the advent of the first serum antibody HIV test in 1985, there has been a need to engage in an appropriate dialogue with patients who undertake HIV testing. The reasons for this are varied, but historically, before the advent of

Advanced Clinical Skills for GU Nurses. Edited by Matthew Grundy-Bowers and Jonathan Davies
© 2007 John Wiley & Sons Ltd

antiretroviral therapy, a diagnosis of HIV was potentially life-threatening, and there was a significant social stigma associated with being HIV-positive. Some may say that this attitude still exists, but in comparison with the 1980s, when HIV-positive children were banned from schools and adults with HIV lost jobs because of their status, much influential work has been done in the UK to change public opinion.

Obtaining verbal or written consent from the patient before taking the test has always been considered best practice. Historically, there have been various methods of obtaining this, but the central importance of having valid consent has always been paramount.

Many groups and individuals have added, adapted and made their own recommendations about the content of pre- and post-test dialogue. Variations have occurred in what is considered good practice in pre- and post-test discussions.

The conversation with the patient regarding HIV testing has over the years been given names such as 'counselling' and 'discussion'. More recently a culture shift has happened within Genito-Urinary Clinics whereby many more individuals are offered HIV testing. This increased emphasis has occurred for a variety of reasons, predominantly related to the increasing rates of HIV infection and the escalating numbers of people in the community who remain undiagnosed. The 2004 figures released from the Health Protection Agency now estimate that there are 53,000 people living in the UK with HIV, and approximately one-third of these are still undiagnosed. In addition, there are increasing numbers of people in the UK who were traditionally seen as having a low prevalence of HIV (such as heterosexuals) who now constitute a significant proportion of the people in this undetected group. As a consequence, one of the main recommendations from the Department of Health publication *The National Strategy for Sexual Health and HIV* is that all patients attending a GUM clinic are offered an HIV test regardless of risk factors, ethnicity or lifestyle.

TESTING FOR HIV

When HIV enters the body, it begins to destroy T4 lymphocyte cells, commonly known as CD4 cells. The host immune system then produces antibodies against the virus. All the commonly used HIV tests look for the presence of HIV antibodies; they do not test for the virus itself.

For routine HIV testing in adults, serum antibody tests are highly reliable and relatively inexpensive. An increasingly popular choice for HIV testing in UK GUM clinics is the rapid antibody test. Blood is taken from patients either with a finger prick sample or by conventional phlebotomy. Trained nurses and medical staff are able to determine in the clinic within a short time-frame (approximately 20 minutes) whether the test for HIV is reactive, thus indicating possible HIV infection. It is more expensive than the traditional laboratory-based serological tests, but as it can take up to one week to obtain results from standard ELISA / Western Blot testing, the rapid antibody test has become more popular in those patients deemed to be within a 'high risk' category. It is also beneficial for patients, as many find the few days of waiting time to be a difficult emotional experience.

Urine and saliva both contain very low concentrations of HIV, and are therefore low-risk transmissible body fluids. However, tests have been developed to detect the presence of HIV antibodies in these fluids, although these tests are not commonly performed in the UK.

WHY DO WE NEED TO PERFORM AN HIV PRE-TEST DISCUSSION?

Primarily the function of performing an HIV pre-test discussion is to obtain informed consent. Patients have a right to information about the implications of HIV testing and they need to make the decision themselves about whether or not to test. The amount of information given to each patient will vary, according to factors such as risk behaviour, and the patient's own wishes. Patients may need more information to make an informed decision about an investigation for a condition, which, if present, could have serious implications for the patient's employment, and/or social or personal life.

Discussing other details, such as how long the test will take and the practicalities of the procedures involved, such as blood or finger-prick sampling, are also important. Where applicable, details of costs or charges that the patient may have to meet, particularly if he/she is not resident in the UK, may also be important to mention, depending on local clinic protocols. These could all be factors in the patient declining an HIV test.

It has also been suggested that a well-performed HIV pre-test discussion may help the patients prepare themselves appropriately for either a positive or a negative diagnosis. Patients may have misconceptions about risk behaviour, and may be mistaken in thinking that they are at either high or low risk.

When providing any information about HIV-testing in a pre-test discussion it is important to find out about patients' individual needs and priorities. For example, patients' beliefs, culture, or occupation may have a bearing on the information they need in order to reach a decision. You should not make assumptions about patients' views, but discuss these matters with them, and ask them whether they have any concerns about the test or the potential risks it may involve. You should provide patients with appropriate information, which should include an explanation of any risks to which they may attach particular significance. Always ask the patient whether they have understood the information and whether they would like more before making a decision.

You must abide by patients' decisions on these issues.

HIV PRE-TEST DISCUSSION

The following guidance is compliant with good practice recommendations and guidelines published by the Department of Health (DH), the British Association for Sexual Health and HIV (BASHH), the British Association of HIV and Aids (BHIVA) and the Society for Sexual Health Advisors (SSHA).

The HIV pre-test discussion has four main functions. The first of these is to assess an individual's previous and current/ongoing risk of acquiring HIV. It can also function as a platform to educate sexually active people about their level of risk in order to avoid only future acquisition of HIV. Moreover, it can help to manage the psychological anxieties arising from the fear and knowledge of HIV. In addition, it can also normalise the process of HIV testing within the context of a sexual health screen, thereby reducing the stigma associated with HIV testing and HIV-positive people.

There are two main elements that make up the HIV pre-test discussion. They can be broken down into the clinician's assessment of risk, and the procedures undertaken while conducting the interview.

TRAINING

An organised training programme should be undertaken before attempting pre- and post-test discussions with patients. The training programme should involve theoretical as well as practical training, followed by an assessment at the end with a trainer. A good programme should always include the following:

* The principles of sexual history-taking
* HIV risk assessment
* The HIV pre-test discussion
* The HIV post-test discussion

HIV RISK ASSESSMENT

An HIV risk assessment should be undertaken on all patients who attend a sexual health clinic for a primary sexual health screen and at each subsequent visit. This assessment should still be undertaken even if the offer of an HIV test has been declined. Most clinics have an HIV pre-test discussion as part of the standard sexual history-taking proforma. However, there remains a need to be well-versed in the questions that are required and the information that should be given to the patient.

One of the aims of the pre-test discussion risk assessment is that the clinician should attempt to establish the likelihood of the patient testing HIV-positive. Some GUM clinics in the United Kingdom have protocols whereby all high-risk patients are referred straight to either Health Advisers or Clinical Nurse Specialists to carry out the HIV pre-test discussion. Different criteria may apply regarding referrals to these professionals; these often depend on patients' risk behaviour and ethnicity. Patients who may be referred include men who have sex with men, intravenous drug users, and people from sub-Saharan Africa or the Caribbean, in addition to people who have sex with people from these groups. In some clinics the person taking the sexual history and assessing symptoms will do the pre-test counselling, and these people tend to be the Nurse Practitioners, Doctors, Health Practitioners or Health Advisers. All these groups should receive training and support about how to conduct appropriate pre- and post-test discussions.

ESTIMATED EXPOSURE RISKS

MEN WHO HAVE SEX WITH MEN (MSM)

When working out the patient's risk factors there are many pertinent questions to be asked. It is important to remember that MSM remain the group at greatest risk of acquiring HIV infection within the UK, accounting for an estimated 84 per cent of infections diagnosed in 2003 (data: HPA). The impact of HIV on MSM in the UK has been profound: 31,430 MSM have been reported as HIV-positive, of whom 12,460 have progressed to AIDS; of these, 9,693 died. Improved survival since the advent of effective antiretroviral therapy in the past decade, with sustained numbers of new HIV diagnoses, has led to increasing numbers of MSM living with diagnosed HIV infection. In the UK it was estimated that, at the end of 2003, just under half (46 per cent, 24,500/53,000) of all HIV infections among adults were among MSM. Furthermore, 26 per cent (6,400) of MSM were unaware of their infection, accounting for 45 per cent of the estimated 14,300 undiagnosed prevalent infections. Data from the Enhanced Syphilis Surveillance programme, collected between April 2001 and September 2004, indicate that 53 per cent (558/1,048) of MSM diagnosed with syphilis in London were known to have co-infection with HIV.

BLACK AND OTHER MINORITY ETHNIC GROUPS

The UK's black and ethnic minority populations continue to be disproportionately affected by poor sexual health. The groups affected and their experiences of HIV and STIs vary greatly, reflecting the diversity present in the migratory patterns, socio-economic circumstances, and experiences of disadvantage and discrimination in these populations. Variation in the incidence of STIs among black and ethnic minority groups is further influenced by several factors, including diverse sexual attitudes and behaviours, patterns of sexual mixing, and differential access to sexual health services. Both the prevalence of heterosexually acquired HIV infections in the UK, including those among pregnant women, and the numbers of new HIV diagnoses reflect the focus of the pandemic in sub-Saharan African countries with close links to the UK. In England, Wales and Northern Ireland, of the HIV-infected heterosexual patients receiving care in 2003 (and for whom ethnicity was reported), 70 per cent were black-African. Over two-fifths of the HIV-infected heterosexuals receiving care reside and are treated outside London; most of these are black-African. Among women who were born in sub-Saharan Africa and who subsequently gave birth in the UK, an estimated one in 42 were HIV-infected in 2003. However, the transmission of HIV from mother to child in the UK has been reduced greatly since the universal offer and recommendation of HIV testing in pregnancy was introduced. Despite this, undiagnosed HIV infection and late diagnosis of longstanding HIV infection continue to be a feature of the treatment histories of black-African men and women, particularly among those attending GUM clinics outside London. Of women born in sub-Saharan Africa attending eight GUM clinics outside London in England, Wales and Northern Ireland, one in 10 had a previously undiagnosed HIV infection.

INJECTING DRUG USERS (IDU)

In addition to laboratory and clinicians' reports there are also data on the prevalence of hepatitis C, hepatitis B, and HIV from the Unlinked Anonymous Prevalence Monitoring Programme Survey of HIV and Hepatitis in Injecting Drug Users. Overall HIV infection remains relatively rare among IDUs in the UK although there is evidence of ongoing and possibly increased transmission. The prevalence of HIV among IDUs has remained substantially higher in London than the rest of the country. Needle- and syringe-sharing increased in the late 1990s, and since then has been stable, with around one in three IDUs reporting this activity in the last month. The sharing of other injecting equipment is more common, whilst few IDUs wash their hands or swab injecting sites prior to injecting. Over 4,000 reported cases of HIV occur in the population of intravenous drug users and this accounts for 6.5 per cent of HIV diagnosis up to 2003.

SEX WITH A KNOWN HIV-POSITIVE PARTNER

The risks associated with individual unprotected sexual exposure with an HIV-positive partner are shown below: these are the estimated risk per incident with someone who is HIV-positive, and may help the clinician in discussing the risk to the index patient. In addition to the factors discussed below (Table 4) the risk of transmission may also be affected by the integrity of the anogenital epithelium and the presence of sexually transmissible infections. The risk per act is probably higher for an individual with multiple HIV-positive partners than it is for those in monogamous relationships.

It is not necessary always to discuss these figures with a patient, although if patients do ask questions about transmission risk, they may be used at your discretion. It is important that if you are using these figures in the pre-test discussion they are put into an appropriate context, and it is emphasised that these are only theoretical risks. They are of more use for the clinician, as they can act as a guide to the likelihood of infection.

SEROCONVERSION

Seroconversion usually occurs between 1 and 10 weeks after the onset of the acute primary exposure to HIV. If a patient is potentially seroconverting, i.e. has had a recent high-risk exposure (Table 4) and has indicative symptoms (Table 5) then a full physical examination and appropriate serological testing should be undertaken; the patient should be handed over to the most senior doctor on duty, depending on the local clinic protocol. This acute primary seroconversion illness is self-limiting, and clinical recovery virtually always occurs.

Approximately 50–80 per cent of patients contracting HIV infection have an acute seroconversion illness – however, most go undiagnosed. Treatment starting at the seroconversion stage (with antiretroviral drugs) may be very beneficial in the longer term in preventing damage to the immune system, as seroconversion illness is known to be associated with more rapid HIV disease progression (Tyrer *et al.*, 2003). It is important to distinguish between seroconversion illnesses, and symptomatic HIV infection. Individuals have their own host responses to HIV, which may or may not lead to symptomatic disease. HIV can remain asymptomatic, potentially for many years. During the early asymptomatic phase, the CD4 lymphocyte count recovers from its initial depression during the primary illness, and may remain at close to normal levels for a number of years before there is a progressive decline associated with the clinical manifestations of HIV disease.

Table 4 Estimated exposure risks

Type of exposure	Risk
Percutaneous exposure	1:333
Mucous membrane exposure	1:1000
Skin exposure	<1:1000
Insertive anal intercourse	1:333
Receptive anal intercourse	1:30–1:125
Receptive vaginal intercourse	1:600–1:2000
Insertive vaginal intercourse	1:1000–1:5000
Intravenous needle/works sharing	1:150

It is vital to remember that some of the symptoms of anxiety may also be attributed to seroconversion (see the section on HIV anxiety below). If you are in any doubt refer the patient to a Clinical Health Psychology department or discuss with an appropriate clinician, Health Practitioner or Health Adviser before undertaking the HIV test.

The patient may be at increased risk of HIV transmission if the contact has a high viral load (i.e. is seroconverting or is in the later stages of the disease). The symptoms of HIV seroconversion are listed in Table 5 below:

Table 5 Symptoms of seroconversion

Symptoms found in >50% patients who are seroconverting	% of patients seroconverting who experience these symptoms
Fever >38°C	77%
Fatigue	66%
Erythematous maculopapular rash	56%
Myalgia	55%
Headache	51%
Symptoms found in 20% to 50% of patients who are seroconverting	% of patients serocoverting who experience these symptoms
Axillary lymphadenopathy	24%
Weight loss	24%
Nausea	24%
Diarrhoea	23%
Night sweats	22%
Cough	22%
Anorexia	21%
Inguinal lymphadenopathy	20%
Symptoms found in 5% to 20% of patients who are seroconverting	% of patients seroconverting who experience these symptoms
Abdominal pain	19%
Oral candidiasis	17%
Vomiting	12%
Photophobia	12%
Sore eyes	12%
Genital ulcer	7%
Tonsillitis	7%
Depression	6%
Dizziness	6%

HIV/AIDS ANXIETY

Some patients who attend a GUM clinic may voice their fears about their possible exposure to HIV infection. These fears can often reveal a misunderstanding of the routes of transmission and the level of risk involved in various sexual and non-sexual situations.

Most commonly anxieties within this group relate to non-sexual modes of spread, such as sharing toothbrushes, cooking and eating utensils, towels and linen, and bathrooms, and non-sexual touching and kissing.

Patients who are worried about such contact usually respond positively to clear, rational discussion about the known routes of transmission and the absence of risk associated with such activities. If their anxiety persists, consideration should be given regarding referral to other services. These patients are often termed the 'worried well'.

THE WORRIED WELL

In using this term it is important to distinguish between a patient who is mildly or justifiably anxious because of reasonable risks as opposed to the patient who is unreasonably worried about exposure to HIV. Only after physical illness has been excluded can the patient be defined as 'worried' and 'well'.

This group of patients can be difficult to manage. Patients in this group can present with multiple physical complaints, which they have interpreted as evidence of their HIV infection. This may occur despite repeated assurances that, on the basis of their history, they could not, (or would be extremely unlikely to), have come into contact with HIV.

Occasionally fears of the infection reach obsessive proportions, and frank obsessive states are often seen in these patients. HIV seems to act as a vehicle for the expression of their psychological vulnerability and sexual guilt.

It is vital to establish the nature and background of their concerns, so that a decision can be made on what the most appropriate intervention would be.

With this group of patients it is important not to propagate their anxiety. It may often be an idea to involve other professionals from disciplines, such as clinical psychology. HIV testing would not be advisable in these cases, pending further psychological assessment. Common characteristics of the 'worried well' include:

- Low-risk sexual activity
- Repeated negative HIV tests
- Multiple symptoms that are misinterpreted, such an features usually associated with undiagnosed viral or postviral (although NOT HIV) infection or anxiety or depression

- High levels of anxiety, depression and obsessional disturbance
- Psychiatric history or a high level of consultations with GPs or other physicians
- Social isolation
- Dependence in close relationships
- Increased potential for suicidal tendencies
- Poor post-adolescent sexual adjustment.

HIV POST-EXPOSURE PROPHYLAXIS (PEP)

Although preventing exposure to HIV remains paramount, evidence suggests that where significant exposure occurs then prompt treatment with combinations of antiretroviral drugs decreases the risk of HIV seroconversion. Although unproven, the presumed mechanism for HIV PEP is that shortly after an exposure to HIV a window period exists. If antiretroviral medications are given they may help to diminish or end viral replication. No definitive data exist on the efficacy of PEP following exposure to HIV other than for occupational exposure. Studies on people with occupational exposure to HIV and animal studies have, however, shown that PEP is effective if commenced as soon as the person is exposed. If there is a delay before the exposed patient presents for PEP, it is usual practice to offer PEP up to 72 hours after exposure. However, its efficacy is likely to fall with increasing delay.

The clinician should make a risk assessment urgently. If the patient is deemed suitable for PEP a senior doctor must assess them as soon as possible. The rationale for PEP varies from clinic to clinic, and it is good practice to have a local clinic protocol for PEP. Further information about PEP can be obtained from BASHH and BHIVA (Walsh & Weston, 2005).

INFORMED CONSENT

All HIV testing should be done with the patient's knowledge and informed consent; this should be free of coercion. Informed consent means that individuals are given enough information about the entire social, legal, health and personal implications of a test to be able to make a fully informed decision to take the test. Ideally, patients must be able to arrive at rational conclusions on the basis of the information given, whilst reconciling this with their current personal circumstances, and make their own decision as to whether they should test at that particular time or defer testing. However, the health benefits of an infected individual's being aware of their HIV status cannot be overestimated. Further information on consent can be obtained from the DH (1996). The key considerations when obtaining consent from a patient for an HIV test are (GMC, 1998):

- The patient must be *competent* to consent.
- The patient needs to *understand* the purpose, risks, harms and benefits of being tested and those of not being tested.
- The patient must consent *voluntarily*.

PRE-TEST DISCUSSION PROCEDURE POINTS

The procedure can be modified depending on the assessment of the patient's previous knowledge and any documented discussion from previous testing. If the same person has previously undertaken pre-test counselling with the patient, it may not be necessary to go over all the points again, but it would be advisable to do so if some time has passed since the patient last attended.

The points that are relevant for discussion with the patient are the following and should generally follow a similar questioning order:

1. If the patient is requesting an HIV test, establish the reason for requesting the test and the possible risk of exposure to HIV. If offering an HIV test as part of an STI screen, explain the rationale for testing and establish the possible risk of exposure to HIV.
2. Establish the patient's knowledge about HIV and the difference between HIV and AIDS; about principles of transmission and prevention strategies and about risk factors.
3. Discuss the pros and cons of testing, including treatment options.
4. Explain the practicalities of taking the test.
5. Explain the relevance of the 3-month window period: i.e. antibody development and the need for repeat testing if the patient falls within this period.
6. Explain the confidentiality within the clinic and clinic records and that GPs are not routinely informed (unless this is requested by a patient). Notes in most GU clinics are kept within the clinic.
7. Explain the meaning of negative, positive and equivocal/ indeterminate results.
8. Discuss the legal, social and psychological implications of a positive result. Explain the issues around insurance companies and testing. The ABI (Association of British Insurers – www.abi.org.uk) has recently confirmed that having had an HIV test will not lead to penalties against individuals applying for life assurance or mortgages. However, failing to disclose a positive HIV test result when applying for a life insurance or mortgage constitutes fraud, and could result in the policy being terminated. Additionally, companies may ask if an HIV test result is pending.
9. Assess the patient's ability to cope with a positive result, including their social support networks. What would the patient do if the result were

positive? Who would they tell? Who would be supportive? How do they usually handle bad news? Be aware of self-harm behaviours such as alcohol and drug abuse.

10. Enquire again if the patient is happy to have an HIV test done today.
11. Explain how HIV results are obtained in your clinic.

ORGANISING HIV RESULTS

The National Strategy for Sexual Health and HIV (DH, 2001) recommends that all new patients attending a GUM clinic are offered an HIV test, with the goal of reducing newly acquired HIV infection by 25 per cent by 2007, as well as reducing waiting times for urgent appointments. This poses a real challenge to current GUM services; if more HIV testing is undertaken, it follows that increased counselling is necessary. This obviously lengthens clinic appointments, and may actually lead to further delays in seeing urgent appointments.

Some GUM clinics now operate a 'no news is good news' policy with patients. This is offered to patients who are deemed to be at low risk of a sexually transmitted infection. This means that within a defined time-period staff from the clinic will only contact the patients if any results come back as being positive, in order to cut down on unnecessary appointments for both patients and clinic staff. Before implementing this policy, it is obviously vital to have a thorough results administration procedure in place, with all test results being checked routinely on all patients that attend. HIV-positive results should never be given over the telephone or by post. Recall for patients who test positive for HIV, if they fail to attend for their results, should only be done by mail. A standardized letter should be sent informing the patient that they missed their appointment and requesting them to return to collect their results.

A clinic appointment should, however, be made for the following reasons:

- The patient is only having an HIV test done and no other screening tests. However, if a patient requests an HIV test only and they are at risk of other STIs, it is best practice to encourage them to have a full sexual health screen. If they still decline you should offer syphilis IgM/IgG, a hepatitis screen (if appropriate) and a *Chlamydia* urine test.
- The patient is a high-risk patient, and there is a strong likelihood that they will be positive.
- The patient is 'anxious' and wants to come back to the clinic to collect their results.
- The patient has limited understanding of English and needs to return to the clinic with an interpreter to discuss the results.

HIV POST-TEST DISCUSSION

GIVING A NEGATIVE HIV RESULT

When disclosing a negative test result, you should explain what the test result means, answer any questions, address the patient's emotional response, and discuss strategies for remaining HIV-negative. It is important not to add any emotional weight to giving a negative result, such as 'the good news is that your HIV result is negative', as you are unaware if this result is good news for the patient or not.

When giving negative test results, remind patients that the results may not be accurate if the client has engaged in behaviours that put him or her at risk during the three months before testing or since the test was done. If appropriate, clients should be offered a repeat test at an appropriate time in the future.

GIVING AN EQUIVOCAL OR INDETERMINATE HIV RESULT

An equivocal or indeterminate result is where laboratory testing from a patient's first blood sample is neither positive nor negative. The tests have differing 'cut off' points, and the virologist performing the test may comment on the *likely* outcome of the test. In this case, communication with the virology department is important, and it may be helpful to impart to the virologist the patient's current health status (any recent seroconversion-type illnesses, risk factors, etc.). You should then document the outcome of this discussion in the patient's notes.

An equivocal HIV result is an uncommon outcome from a serum antibody test, and can be a difficult result to give to a patient. It can be complicated for the result-giver to explain and difficult for the patient to understand. It may be especially complicated if the patient has heightened anxiety levels regarding the result of their HIV blood test. It is usually necessary that extra time during the consultation should be allocated for the result-giver to answer questions and explain the meaning of this test result.

Post-test discussion points when giving an equivocal HIV result

1. Inform the patient clearly of the nature of the equivocal HIV result and what this result means.
2. Give the patient the opportunity to read the result, pointing out the clinic number and date of birth.
3. Clarify the patient's understanding of the result.
4. Explain the need for a further blood specimen on the day of receiving the result for repeat testing, which may provide a more conclusive result.

5. Give clear guidance, based on your laboratory's information of when the next serum results will be available, and arrange an appointment for the patient to return.
6. Assess and address the patient's immediate reactions. Most equivocal results do turn out to be negative, but it is important to check the history and the nature of the risk, and the timing of the last risk activity.
7. Offer further support if the patient requires it.

GIVING AN HIV-POSITIVE TEST RESULT

When giving an HIV-positive result, remember that it is a medical diagnosis. It is essential that positive results are not dealt with single-handedly. They require a multidisciplinary approach, so that the patient is seen promptly and the service is responsive to their needs both physically and mentally. Depending on local clinic services, and the patient's health and mental status, you may need immediately to involve a senior doctor, HIV clinical nurse specialists, TB nurse specialists, clinical psychologists, health advisers and health practitioners.

Once you are in a private consultation room and the confirmation of ID and introductions have been made do not delay in giving the result to the patient. Often our faces and body language are our biggest give-away, and, if the patient is attuned to this then they may pick up that something is not right with their results from the expression on your face or your body language from the moment you call them in. There is no easy way of breaking bad news, and the best way to do this is to be honest. Different patient reactions require different responses from you. You should not show any 'over the top' emotions on your part. Sometimes it may be appropriate to wait for the patient to speak before you say anything else immediately after telling them the result. In some clinics it is practice that the patients see the Health Adviser immediately after the result is given (SSHA, 2004).

Post-test discussion points when giving an HIV-positive result

1. Inform the patient of the nature of the HIV result clearly, and what this result means.
2. Give the patient the opportunity to read the result, pointing out the clinic number and date of birth.
3. Clarify the patient's understanding of the result.
4. Address the patient's immediate reactions. Each patient will receive the news in his or her own way. Ensure there is time for discussion of immediate concerns. Find out what the patient will be doing in the next 24–48 hours.
5. Offer further support if the patient requires it.
6. Carry out an assessment of any social or mental health issues.
7. Discuss the need for further blood tests to assess health status and a repeat test for confirmation.

8. Refer for specialist management, including treatment where appropriate. Depending on your clinic's practices this may involve an HIV appointment with a specialist HIV doctor and clinical nurse specialist to discuss the results of further tests and give the patient an appointment card confirming the dates and times.
9. Check if the patient has any immediate medical problems. In the event of any symptoms, an immediate link with a doctor is indicated.
10. Offer follow-up appointments and ongoing support for the patient, partner and/or family.
11. Find out who the patient may tell, and clarify available support systems.
12. Clarify transmission issues, and how patients can minimise risk to themselves and others.
13. Give details of support services and resource material.
14. Give the patient written details of the ways s/he can contact the health adviser, and help-line numbers, for example the National AIDS Helpline.
15. Raise partner notification. It may be appropriate to address partner notification issues in the immediate post-test session. Patients will often raise partner notification at this point themselves.

RECOGNISING PATIENTS' ANXIETIES

Most patients who test positive for HIV are likely to have a high degree of anxiety, even before getting their results. The reasons for this may be varied, but generally they may involve knowing people who have already died from AIDS-related illnesses, misconceptions about the facts of HIV infection, and anxieties about informing close family and partners.

While giving a result, you should be aware that the anxiety and emotion that accompany a positive result are likely to have a significant effect on the patient, and they normally need some time to absorb the initial result before you give them any further information. With most patients, it is generally advised not to give small amounts of information about specific areas (e.g. viral loads and CD4 counts), and to focus more on how the patient is, who they are going to inform about the result and who will be able to give them some emotional support if needed. At a follow-up appointment in a week's time, normally when they return for the confirmatory second HIV test and other blood-test results, it may be more appropriate to go into further details about the infection.

TALKING ABOUT PATIENTS' PROGNOSES

When discussing HIV infection with newly diagnosed patients, it can be difficult to work out a balance between giving factual and practical information, whilst simultaneously giving the patient hope for the future.

It is common for patients to ask questions such as 'How many years will I live for?' after learning of the infection. Honesty and pragmatism are essential when discussing a patient's prognosis, but a realistic optimism should be applied whenever appropriate.

Whilst recognising the seriousness of the diagnosis, you should avoid speculating about a patient's life expectancy, stressing that each individual case is different and that strategies to extend survival and new treatment therapies are being developed and tested at a rapid pace. The fact that they are diagnosed in a first world country will mean that treatment options are readily available and expert care is available.

REFERRAL TO AN HIV SPECIALIST DOCTOR AND ASSOCIATED SPECIALISTS IF HIV-POSITIVE

Now that the HIV result has been given and confirmed, the next step in working with this patient is to refer them appropriately. Most GUM clinics have specialist services such as HIV physicians, and other associated specialists in HIV. Depending on the area in which you work you may be able to refer newly diagnosed patients directly into these services, or you may need to contact them and refer in another way. Some patients may prefer to have their HIV care moved to another clinic, which in most cases can be organised by your service by means of writing a referral letter once a confirmatory HIV test has been reported. A policy should be set up in every area that takes and gives HIV results. It should detail the steps that need to occur in dealing with a new positive diagnosis and onward referral. If such documentation does not exist it is a good idea to contact a GUM clinic near to your service and ask for some guidance.

REFERRAL FOR COUNSELLING AND OTHER SERVICES IF HIV-POSITIVE OR -NEGATIVE

Newly diagnosed patients may require immediate assistance in attaining additional counselling for emotional distress, peer support, assistance with financial concerns, future planning, child-care issues, housing, or other practical concerns. Such patients may also require referrals to services related to family planning. Where available, you should refer patients to appropriate community organisations, social agencies, peer support groups, and other resources near to the area in which they live or work. However, some patients may wish to travel further afield.

Patients who test negative may also require referrals to family planning, healthcare, counselling, or social services. All patients, positive and negative, should be provided with condoms, counselling on prevention, and information about where to obtain additional condoms.

CONCLUSION

Many resources are available to add to your knowledge in pre- and post-test HIV discussion. As with many things, a mixture of theory, supervised discussion and practice is the best way to become proficient in these skills. My best advice is to always remain open-minded about the patient's response to the result you are giving and never assume a particular reaction to a result. That way you will hopefully never be caught off guard, and your response, whether verbal or non-verbal, will hopefully never be inappropriate.

The other thing I would like to stress is, that there is no easy way of breaking bad news. Many of us still find the process difficult, even after years of giving positive and negative HIV results, especially when dealing with certain groups in which the result is unexpected, such as with a very young person. Always discuss the process, if it is difficult, as soon as possible with your supervisor or a work colleague.

REFERENCES

DH (Department of Health) (2001) Better prevention, better services better sexual health – The National Strategy for Sexual Health & HIV. DH: London

GMC (General Medical Council) (1998) Seeking Patients' Consent: The Ethical Considerations, November. GMC, London

Pratt R (2003) *HIV EAIDS: A Foundation for Nursing and Healthy Strategy for Nursing Care*, 5th edn. Edward Arnold, London

Shorter Oxford Dictionary, 3rd edn (1994) Oxford University Press, Oxford.

SSHA (Society for Sexual Health Advisors) (2004) *The Manual For Sexual Health Advisors*, OH, London

Tyrer F, Walker AS, Gillett J, Porter K *et al.* (2003) 'The relationship between HIV seroconversion illness, HIV test interval and time to AIDS in a seroconverter cohort.' *Epidemiological Infections* 2003 Dec;131(3):1117–23

Walsh J, Weston R (2005) 'Clinical Guidance for the Management of Post Exposure Prophylaxis (PEP) Following Occupational & Non-Occupational Exposure of Adults to HIV-1 & Other Human Retroviruses.' St Marys Hospital Policy, London

9 Health Promotion and Sexual Health

DEBBY PRICE

INTRODUCTION

Health promotion is an essential aspect of the role of all health and social care professionals engaged in sexual health work. The vital nature of sexual health promotion is highlighted by the fact that the unintentional consequences of sexual health behaviour are almost always preventable; for example, sexually transmitted infections (STIs) or unintended pregnancy. However, the promotion of sexual health has a broader role in helping individuals achieve good health and well-being. This chapter aims to provide a theoretical framework to help clarify the purpose of interventions designed to improve the health of clients accessing sexual health services. While the emphasis of the chapter will be on sexual health promotion, it is important to recognise that those involved in sexual health work are often in a prime position to engage in other health-promotion activities covering a wide range of topics, including healthy eating, smoking cessation, drugs and alcohol and assertiveness skills, some of which are inextricably linked with sexual health behaviour.

Format of chapter:

- Defining what we mean by health and sexual health
- Defining what we mean by health promotion and its relationship with public health
- Sexual health promotion strategies
- Challenges to sexual health promotion.

WHAT IS HEALTH?

Before exploring what we mean by health promotion it is important to clarify what is meant by the term 'health'. It has been some time since the World Health Organisation offered their definition of health as: '*a state of complete physical, mental and social well-being, and not merely the absence of disease*'

Advanced Clinical Skills for GU Nurses. Edited by Matthew Grundy-Bowers and Jonathan Davies
© 2007 John Wiley & Sons Ltd

(WHO, 1946). This statement was radical at the time in that it acknowledged that health was more than merely the absence of disease, but encompassed social and psychological dimensions too. It is a statement that is arguably relevant today, though the definition has many critics, including Ewles and Simnet (2003), who argue that the definition is both 'unrealistic' and 'static'. More recently the WHO has further debated the concept of health, and proposes:

> ... a conception of health as the extent to which an individual or group is able, on the one hand, to realize aspirations and satisfy needs; and, on the other hand, to change or cope with the environment. Health is, therefore, seen as a resource for everyday life, not the objective of living; it is a positive concept emphasizing social and personal resources, as well as physical capacities (WHO 1984, cited in Ewles and Simnett, 2003).

The definition offered here is perhaps a much wider examination of health and looks at 'health' from a different perspective, considering health as an element of life rather than as the sole objective of living.

So do these broader health definitions sit comfortably within the sphere of sexual health or are they limiting definitions that may exclude aspects of sexual health care? Certainly this definition is useful when considering sexual health in that it suggests that it is important for individuals and groups to be helped to realise their full potential and satisfy their needs. It is important that we now define what we mean by sexual health.

WHAT IS SEXUAL HEALTH?

A good starting-point is the World Health Organisation's (WHO) definition of sexual health outlined below:

> Sexual health is a state of physical, emotional, mental and social well-being in relation to sexuality; it is not merely the absence of disease, dysfunction or infirmity. Sexual health requires a positive and respectful approach to sexuality and sexual relationships, as well as the possibility of having pleasurable and safe sexual experiences, free of coercion, discrimination and violence. For sexual health to be attained and maintained, the sexual rights of all persons must be respected, protected and fulfilled (WHO, 2002 internet).

In this definition the WHO strives to acknowledge the complexities of sexual relationships and the importance of respect and consideration for others in achieving individual sexual health. In considering absence of disease, freedom from coercion and violence and respect of all persons the definition allows us to consider sexual health from a human perspective. This definition is important in that it recognises the gender and power conflicts that exist in sexual relationships and also the diversity of human beings and their sexual orientations and choices.

More recently the Department of Health (DH) has similarly proposed that sexual health is an important part of physical and mental health and that it is a *'key part of our identity as human beings together with the fundamental rights to privacy, family life and living free from discrimination'* (DH, 2001).

The WHO also gives consideration to sexual rights that should be an integral part of any discussion considering how people can achieve sexual health.

SEXUAL RIGHTS

Sexual rights embrace human rights that are already recognised in national laws, international human rights documents and other consensus statements.

They include the right of all persons, free of coercion, discrimination and violence, to:

* attain the highest accessible standard of sexual health, including access to sexual and reproductive healthcare services;
* seek, receive and impart information related to sexuality;
* receive sexuality education;
* receive respect for bodily integrity;
* choose their partner;
* decide to be sexually active or not;
* practice consensual sexual relations;
* practice consensual marriage;
* decide whether or not, and when, to have children; and
* pursue a satisfying, safe and pleasurable sexual life.

In achieving sexual rights consideration must be given to the responsible exercise of human rights requiring that all persons respect the rights of others (WHO, 2002 internet).

SEXUAL HEALTH: A GLOBAL PANDEMIC AND A NATIONAL PUBLIC HEALTH ISSUE

In 1995 the WHO conducted a study that estimated at least 33 million cases of curable STIs had occurred during that year. The crucial thing about this statistic was that these STIs were not only curable but preventable, and their complications ranked among the top 10 causes of healthy days lost by adults in the developing world (WHO, 1995).

Nationally in the UK, sexual health has been high on successive governments' agendas for improvement in response to the rise in sexually transmitted infections and a poor record in teenage pregnancy. The British government clearly sees sexual health as being a key health issue, identifying the following consequences of poor sexual health:

- Pelvic inflammatory disease, which can cause ectopic pregnancies and infertility
- HIV
- Cervical and other genital cancers
- Hepatitis, chronic liver disease and liver cancer
- Recurrent genital herpes
- Bacterial vaginosis and premature delivery
- Unintended pregnancy and abortions
- Psychological consequences of sexual coercion and abuse
- Poor educational, social and economic opportunities for teenage mothers

(DH, 2001).

So, what is the government responding to? In 2005 was there really a crisis in the sexual health of the nation? To answer these questions perhaps we should briefly examine the statistics provided by the Health Protection Agency (HPA) and the Office of National Statistics (ONS) to give a clear picture of the current status of sexually transmitted infections and teenage pregnancy in the UK recently.

SEXUALLY TRANSMITTED INFECTIONS

Recent statistics recording the number of new diagnoses of sexually transmitted infections between 2003 and 2004 in England and Wales show the following:

- An overall rise in the number of new diagnoses seen in GUM clinics of 2 per cent in 2004 compared to 2003 (from 735,302 in 2003 to 751,282 in 2004).
- *Chlamydia* increased by 8 per cent (from 95,879 in 2003 to 103,932 in 2004).
- Syphilis increased by 37 per cent (from 1641 in 2003 to 2252 in 2004).
- Genital warts increased by 4 per cent (from 76,457 in 2003 to 79,618 in 2004).
- Gonorrhoea decreased by 10 per cent (from 24,915 in 2003 to 22,320 in 2004).
- Genital herpes decreased by 1 per cent (from 19,180 in 2003 to 18,923 in 2004).

(HPA, October 2005)

These figures demonstrate a small but significant increase in reported sexually transmitted infections between 2003 and 2004 (with the exception of syphilis, which had a more significant rise). However, there has been a downturn in the infection rates for gonorrhea and genital herpes.

In order better to understand the current problems it is helpful to examine the figures over a wider time-period.

Table 6 below is an illustration of the same set of sexually transmitted infections studied over a nine-year period. This bigger picture offers a better

Table 6 Health Protection Agency October 2005

	2004	% change 2003–2004	% change 1995–2004
Chlamydia	103,932	+8%	222%
Genital warts	79,618	+4%	32%
Gonorrhoea	22,320	−10%	111%
Genital herpes	18,923	−1%	15%
Syphilis	2,252	+37%	1497%

illustration of the scale of the problem faced in the UK. The most worrying statistics demonstrate the return of syphilis into the sexual ill health of the population of the UK, and, of course, the massive increase in rates of diagnosed *Chlamydia*.

In examining these statistics, it is important to acknowledge some of the possible anomalies that may exist in the reporting of Sexually Transmitted Infections:

- The figures only represent cases diagnosed and reported by Genito-urinary Medicine Clinics in England and Wales. There are other opportunities for testing and treatment within the healthcare system that do not contribute to the reported figures.
- These are only the cases that are reported. Many infections can be asymptomatic or confused with other conditions, and consequently we can reasonably assume that actual rates may in fact be higher than the reported rates.
- The increase in reported cases of *Chlamydia* may be down to improved diagnostic technology now picking up infections that have in fact been present for some considerable time.

It is clear, however, that in England and Wales there is currently an epidemic of sexually transmitted infections. The government's response needs to tackle head-on these trends in infection rates through coherent policy strategies and the longer-term modernization of services. Policy-makers and health professionals alike must remain cognisant of the long-term damage caused by sexually transmitted infections, including infertility and a greater risk of contracting HIV. Ignoring the need to tackle STIs may well result in a greater subsequent burden on scarce health resources in the treatment and management of HIV and infertility.

TEENAGE PREGNANCY

Despite the overall trend towards later childbearing, teenage pregnancy rates in England and Wales remain stubbornly high, with nearly 8,000 conceptions among girls under the age of 16 in 2001 (Social Trends 33, 2003). Of these conceptions in 2001, almost 400 were to girls under the age of 14, under half of which led to maternities. There was also a variation across age in the number of legal abortions. In 2002, 61 per cent of conceptions to 14-year-olds resulted in legal abortions, 6 per cent higher than the number in the 15-year-old group, which was the next highest (Social Trends 33, 2003).

To put this in context, throughout most of Western Europe teenage birth rates have fallen rapidly since the 1970s, while in the United Kingdom the rates have remained at the 1980s level or above. In 2001 the United Kingdom had the highest rate of live births to teenage girls in the European Union, with an average of 29 live births per 1000 girls aged 15–19. This was nearly 44 per cent higher than Portugal, the country with the next highest rate. Sweden and Italy had the lowest rates, at around 7 live births per 1000 girls aged 15–19 (Social Trends 33, 2003).

The impact of unintended pregnancy for teenage girls is physical, psychological and social. Births to teenage mothers are particularly likely to take place outside marriage. In 2000 almost 9 in 10 live births to women aged under twenty in England and Wales occurred outside marriage. The report on teenage pregnancy by the Social Exclusion Unit in 1999 identified the impacts of teenage pregnancy as the following:

- Poor antenatal health, lower birthweight babies and higher infant mortality rates
- The health of teenage parents and their children is worse than average
- More likely to be living in poverty
- Disproportionately likely to suffer relationship breakdown
- Their daughters are more likely to become teenage mothers themselves.

ACHIEVING SEXUAL HEALTH: THE ROLE OF HEALTH AND SOCIAL CARE PROFESSIONALS

It can be seen from the above discussion that helping people to achieve sexual health is a vital part of the role of health professionals, but at the same time an extremely challenging one. Health professionals need a range of knowledge and skills to be able to engage with individual clients and groups in the promotion of sexual health. Probably the most crucial is the ability to deal with sensitive, confidential and personal issues and to be able to discuss aspects of clients' lifestyle and behaviours that are not usually shared outside a close sexual relationship. It is important that health professionals involved in sexual health promotion have a broad understanding of the theory and practice of health promotion and the current emphasis being placed on this by the current public health policy agenda.

DEFINING HEALTH PROMOTION

The WHO (1984) defined health promotion as: '*the process of enabling people to increase control over, and to improve their health*'. This provides a good starting-point to any discussion on what we mean by health promotion. The definition encompasses an element of empowerment, but assumes that people have full control over the circumstances in which they live and are able to choose healthy lifestyles freely. This is a vital area of debate in sexual health promotion, as it is often the case that clients do not have full control over their circumstances, owing to the very nature of sexual relationships.

Similarly, Seedhouse (2004) suggests that the concept of health promotion is one that implies enablement, in that health promotion activities provide the foundations to enable the achievement of personal and/or group potential. He proposes that health is achieved by removing obstacles and by providing the means by which chosen goals can be obtained.

Health promotion is generally regarded as an overarching term encompassing a range of activities (Tannahill, 1985; Naidoo and Wills, 1998). Tannahill (1985) argues that the term includes health education and environmental, legal and fiscal measures designed to enhance health. He distinguishes health promotion from curative, technological or acute health services as comprising those activities that are health-enhancing, and proposes a model of health promotion that consists of three overlapping spheres; health education, prevention (of ill health) and health protection. Professionals practising in the sexual health field are often involved in all three spheres of activity.

In a similar way Naidoo and Wills (1998) see health promotion as an umbrella term that encompasses four key activities:

- **Disease prevention,** for example activities focusing on individuals or groups, such as cervical screening.
- **Health education and information** – these are activities that are aimed at preventing disease and enhancing health through education. Examples include sexual health workshops as part of personal and social education in schools, or individual sexual health promotion in a surgery or clinic, or media campaigns to raise public awareness.
- **Public health promotion** – activities that promote health through social and environmental measures.
- **Community development** – activities that enable individuals to develop personal skills, knowledge and personal networks, for example peer education and buddying schemes.

Many theorists argue that health promotion draws on all activities that seek to improve the health of individuals, groups and the wider population. For instance Tones (1990) argues that 'health promotion incorporates all measures designed to promote health and handle disease' and that:

> *A major feature of health promotion is undoubtedly the importance of 'healthy public policy' with its potential for achieving social change via legislation, fiscal, economic and other forms of environmental engineering* (Tones, 1990, p. 3).

In this definition Tones suggests the close relationship between health promotion activity and public health in stressing the importance of public health policy. Certainly it is difficult to discuss health promotion without examining its relationship with the wider sphere of public health. This is essential when considering sexual health promotion, given the recent government public health strategies relating to sexual health, which clearly indicate the need for sexual health promotion with a range of client groups, including teenagers and young adults, gay men and black and ethnic minority groups.

PUBLIC HEALTH

According to Naidoo and Wills (2000) public health is characterised by several factors – a concern for the health of the whole population (whether a geographical population, a client group such as gay men, or a group of people experiencing a specific health problem, such as *Chlamydia*); a concern for the prevention of illness and disease; and, lastly, a recognition of the many social factors that contribute to health.

There are a number of strands to public health.

- Health protection, enabling people to live in a clean, safe environment, or preventing them from contracting diseases by, for example, implementing a needle exchange programme.
- Health promotion, tackling some of the determinants of health such as poverty and unemployment, or implementing specific programmes such as safer sex campaigns. Addressing the issues of poverty and unemployment can be regarded as a structural approach to health promotion through changing the fabric of society; whereas safer sex programmes encompass a behavioural approach, whereby individuals and groups are encouraged to take control of their lives and determine the actions they take.
- Health maintenance, that is, maintaining or preventing further deterioration in health by operationalising screening programmes to identify the early onset of disease – for example cervical screening programmes.

As Naidoo and Wills (2000) point out, public health and health promotion share many principles and strategies. Public health encompasses strands of health protection, health promotion, health maintenance and the provision of health, social and voluntary services to improve population health. Health promotion is the translation of these strategies into practice and raising the awareness of these issues. For example, a public health strategy might be the reduction of teenage pregnancy rates while the health promotion aspect of this strategy might be the development of leaflets for teenagers containing information about safer sex and contraception, the delivery of sex education programmes in schools, and/or a family planning nurse discussing sexual health with teenage clients on a one-to-one basis.

RECENT PUBLIC HEALTH POLICY RELATED TO SEXUAL HEALTH

As a response to the continuing epidemic of sexually transmitted infections and the high teenage pregnancy rate in England and Wales the government has delivered White Papers and guidelines to begin to tackle the problem. These include;

- Social Exclusion Unit report on *Teenage Pregnancy* (Teenage Pregnancy Unit, 1999)
- *The National Strategy for Sexual Health and HIV* (DH, 2001)
- *The National Strategy for Sexual Health and HIV Implementation Action Plan* (DH, 2002)
- *The National Chlamydia Screening Programme in England* (DH, 2004b)
- *Choosing Health: Making Healthier Choices Easier Choices* (DH, 2004a)
- *Recommended Standards for Sexual Health Services* (DH, 2005)

The most significant of these was the publication of *The National Strategy for Sexual Health and HIV* (DH, 2001). This was the first of the major policy documents to concentrate solely on the provision and modernisation of sexual health services. It was also unique in that it examined the related problems of HIV and Sexually Transmitted Infections in the same policy document. The main aims of the strategy are to:

- Reduce the incidence of HIV and STIs;
- Reduce the prevalence of undiagnosed HIV and STIs;
- Reduce unintended pregnancy rates;
- Improve health and social care of people living with HIV; and
- Reduce the stigma associated with HIV and STIs.

It is clear from the strategy document that the approach was one that viewed sexual health as an intergral part of public health and acknowledged that 'sexual health' inequalities exist between different social groups and cultures. The Government proposed that these aims would be met through the following actions:

- The setting of a new target for a 25 per cent reduction of newly acquired HIV and gonorrhoea infections by the end of 2007 (DH, 2001)

- The provision of clear information about sexual health so that people can make informed decisions about preventing STIs and HIV
- Ensuring the provision of a sound evidence base for effective HIV/STI prevention
- The development of managed networks for HIV and sexual health services, leading to a more integrated sexual health service.

Alongside the recommendations of the sexual health strategy the *Teenage Pregnancy* report (Social Exclusion Unit 1999) made recommendations specific to teen pregnancy, including the aim to halve teenage conceptions among under 18s by 2010.

The *Sexual Health* Strategy, along with the *Teenage Pregnancy* report, has been welcomed as an important step in tackling sexual health and integrating sexual health services in England. However, critics are disappointed that it does not go far enough – in particular that the policy was not given the status of a National Service Framework (Alder, 2003; Duffin, 2005).

THE ROLE OF THE HEALTH PROFESSIONAL – PROMOTING SEXUAL HEALTH

Healthcare professionals are vital to the achievement of government sexual health strategies and the improvement of the overall sexual health of the population. For many health professionals the key way in which they can respond to help to achieve Government targets in reducing the prevalence of sexually transmitted infections or reduce unwanted pregnancy is through their health promotion work. Both the *Teenage Pregnancy* report (Social Exclusion Unit, 1999) and the *National Strategy for Sexual* Health (DH, 2001) clearly identify ignorance as being a key factor, with people lacking the information they need to make informed choices that will affect their sexual health (Cooper, 2001). This is an area in which the health promotion skills of health and social care professionals are key to providing accurate, individually tailored information; though as we will see, sexual health promotion is a much more complex business than just providing information.

In order that Government targets are achieved and to move towards a more universal goal of good sexual health for everyone, all health and social care professionals need to respond to the opportunities presented to them to promote the sexual health of their clients and patients. This includes generic professionals such as GPs, practice nurses, teachers and youth workers, as well as dedicated sexual health professionals.

The preceding discussion has highlighted the broad objectives of health promotion in the context of public health, and it can be seen that there are many possible approaches to health-promotion work. The health-promotion approach chosen by practitioners will be dependent on the aims of their health-promotion activity. Ewles and Simnett (2003) suggest that health promoters need to clarify two main health-promotion aims before starting:

- **Whether the aim is to change the individual or to change society**
The choice here is between a traditional approach to health education, which aims to change the behaviour of individuals to induce them to adopt a healthier lifestyle, or a more radical health-promotion approach, which seeks to make the environment and society a healthier place in which to live – to change the structure of society. In other words, professionals need to ask themselves whether the scope of their work is to be focused on individuals (for example, persuading an individual to adopt safer sexual practices) or to be involved in more radical approaches such as campaigning for sexual health-promotion campaigns to be shown on children's television or attempting to change societal attitudes towards gays.

- **Whether the aim is for compliance or informed choice**
Here health promoters need to decide what it is they want to achieve – compliance or informed choice. Professionals need to ask themselves whether the aim of their health-promotion activity is to ensure that the public or a client complies with a health initiative or programme through the use of education, or through media publicity or through persuasion. Or is their aim to create circumstances in which the client or the public are enabled to make informed choices? If so, do their clients have the skills and ability to enact those choices? Many health professionals will say they want to allow clients to make informed choices, but in reality feel uncomfortable when a client chooses the option (or lifestyle behaviour) that is regarded as not being healthy (for example continuing to have unprotected sex)! This is an important dimension, which it is important for all professionals to explore with themselves before embarking on health-promotion work.

It is essential, then, that all professionals working in the sexual health field have a holistic understanding of sexual health and a non-judgemental approach in dealing with clients and patients. Alison Duffin, writing about the role of the nurse in sexual health, argues that nurses need a: '. . . *holistic approach to sexual health which encompasses health promotion advice, recognizes varying sexual health behavior, understands that sexually acquired infection can interfere with sexual function, and most importantly accepts that psychological factors impair and inhibit sexual functioning and relationships*' (Duffin, 2005, p. 417).

Specifically, Ingram Fogel (1990) argues that sexual health promoters need the following skills:

- an accurate knowledge base;
- self-awareness of their own personal value system and self-acceptance as a sexual being; and
- the ability to communicate genuinely and therapeutically with clients.

APPROACHES TO HEALTH PROMOTION

Both Ewles and Simnett (2003) and Naidoo and Wills (2000) suggest that there are five key approaches to health-promotion work, each reflecting different objectives and ways of working. Table 7 explores each of these approaches using examples from sexual health.

DECIDING ON WHICH APPROACH TO USE

Broadly speaking the above approaches fall into two main categories – firstly, those that focus on the individual and, arguably, to be successful require clients to modify their behaviour; and secondly, those methods that employ community-centred/societal change approaches.

Many professionals adopt methods that focus on individual approaches with the aims of improving knowledge and awareness of sexual health issues, encouraging the adoption of healthy or safer patterns of behaviour and encouraging those individuals who continue to be at risk to modify and sustain changes in their sexual behaviour. These approaches are attractive to professionals, as they are seen as achievable within busy work schedules, and certainly do have some advantages, as information can be tailored specifically to individual need.

However, professionals need to be aware of the limitations of these approaches, and in particular the need to guard against 'victim blaming'. The majority of sexual health 'problems', such as sexually transmitted infections or unintended pregnancy, are indeed preventable. However, while this may be true, it is simplistic to go on to assume that individuals are at fault and to blame when things go wrong. This discussion will be expanded further below, when we come to examine the challenges to successful sexual health promotion.

A further limitation of approaches focusing on the individual is the tendency to concentrate on 'medical' models of health promotion such as sexual health screening or preventive treatment. Imrie *et al.* (2005) argue for a more positive approach to health promotion for men who have sex with men than purely concentrating on clinic-based sexual health interventions such as sexual health screening and the treatment of sexually transmitted disease. They point to the fact that many men who have sex with men and who have HIV have a higher prevalence of concurrent psychosocial health problems, including recreational drug use and early childhood sexual abuse, and argue that little has been done to develop and evaluate interventions that address wider behavioural and lifestyle issues.

Mussen *et al.* (1998) suggest that approaches that address broader influences on sexual health may be more fruitful, in that it may be easier to change some of the factors influencing behaviour than to change sexual health behaviour directly. They suggest that health promoters could concentrate on other

Table 7

Approach	Aim	Value system	Health promotion strategy
Medical	To identify those at risk of cervical cancer/ *Chlamydia*.	Expert-led, top-down – passive conforming client.	Early detection and treatment of cervical cancer through cervical screening/*Chlamydia* screening.
Behaviour change	Encourage individuals to take responsibility for their own health and choose healthier lifestyles, e.g. safer sex; using contraception to plan a family.	Expert-led, i.e. healthy lifestyle defined by health promoter.	Persuasion through one-to-one advice, leaflets, school sexual health education.
Educational	To give individuals knowledge, and understanding to enable them to make informed decisions about their health e.g. clients will have an understanding about the effects of unsafe sex on their health and will be able to make an informed decision about whether or not to practise safer sex.	Individual right of free choice. Role of health promoter is to identify educational content.	Giving of information about effects of unsafe sex and not using contraception. Helping clients explore their own values and attitudes and come to a decision, e.g. through one-to-one discussion or small groups. Helping clients to change sexual behaviour if they want to, through acquisition of assertiveness skills.
Empowerment	To work with clients or communities to meet their perceived needs, e.g. working with client asking for help to practise safer sex or woman wanting to space her family.	Client-centred – clients treated as equals. Health promoter is a facilitator. Client becomes empowered.	Client to identify health-promotion issue. Use of negotiation, networking facilitation, e.g. 'buddy' system to support clients to practise safer sex or select most appropriate form of contraception for them.
Social change	To address inequalities in health based on class, race, gender, sexual orientation, geography. Make healthier choices easier choices.	Need to make environment health-enhancing. Entails social regulation top-down approach, e.g. public health legislation, fiscal controls.	Political and social action to change physical and social environment, e.g. clinics and other sexual health services more available for hard-to-reach groups; encouraging greater acceptance of age, gender and ethnic diversity.

Source: Adapted from Ewles and Simnett 2003.

factors, including recognising the influence of peer norms; empowering communities in their prevention efforts; campaigning for better education in schools; or providing access to appropriate information and services, such as the provision of condoms for anal sex.

Alternative approaches, such as sexual health promotion informed by psychosexual counselling models while still focusing on the individual, offer a more positive approach, though they do require more time from the professional. In these approaches the health professional works with the clients to explore the contexts of their lives and relationships and supports them in developing their own personal strategies for sexual health. Abraham and Sheeran (1993) suggest that much sexual activity is not open to negotiation, and therefore sexual skills training, such as training in assertiveness skills, would bring about more effective and empowering change.

Another alternative is to explore community-centred approaches, and there have been good examples in the sexual health promotion field (Watney, 1990; Rhodes, 1990). Rooney and Scott (1992) are very supportive of community action, pointing to the widespread adoption of safer sex and the existence of a supportive and affirmative gay culture providing grassroots community education, and contrast this with the lack of success of individualistic modules of behaviour change. However, Elford et al. (2002) argue that while peer education programmes have been shown to be effective in the United States, they failed to show any significant impact on the risk behaviours of homosexual men in two studies in London and Glasgow.

DISCUSSION – CHALLENGES TO EFFECTIVE HEALTH PROMOTION

Sexual health promotion raises a number of dilemmas for health promoters, which will now be considered.

SEXUAL HEALTH BEHAVIOURS

Professionals working in sexual health promotion need to be cognisant of the way in which sexual health behaviour differs from other health-related behaviour (Mussen et al. 1998). Crucially, an individual's behaviour may have a 'direct, immediate and drastic effect on their partner's sexual health' (Mussen et al. p. 241), whether through infection with HIV or causing an unintended pregnancy. Mussen et al. (1998) argue, though, that the emphasis on, in particular, prevention of HIV has restricted sexual health promotion activity to encouraging people to change their sexual behaviour, and that this has been to the detriment of other activities aimed at improving sexual health in a wider sense, thus improving overall health and well-being.

TARGETING SEXUAL HEALTH PROMOTION

The Government has set specific targets for sexual health promotion (for example teenage pregnancy and STIs), and has identified 'high-risk' groups, such as teenagers, gay men, young adults and black and ethnic minority groups (DH, 1991). However, one of the results of this is that professionals fail to recognise sexual health promotion needs and opportunities in other population groups, such as older newly single heterosexuals. In addition, some government public health strategies, such as *Chlamydia* screening, have excluded men, and this has been criticised by Hart *et al.* (2002), who question the wisdom of such a policy, as men have the same risk of infection from *Chlamydia* as women.

PERCEPTIONS OF RISK

For behaviour change to occur not only does the individual have to understand the message but they also need to believe they are at risk and that behaviour change is therefore worthwhile. Evidence has shown that while health-promotion interventions and campaigns increase people's knowledge of the role of condom use in the prevention of HIV, they have little effect on attitudes and behaviour (McEwan and Bhopal 1991). This is often due to individuals' perceptions that they have a low risk of contracting HIV – this is particularly true of heterosexuals over the age of 35 (HEA, 1994).

A study of the use of the emergency contraceptive pill and sexual risk behaviour investigated participants' perceived risk of HIV, STIs and pregnancy. While the majority of the participants (78 per cent) felt they were at a medium to high risk of pregnancy, 79 per cent felt they were at little or no risk of HIV and 68 per cent at little or no risk of STIs (Dupont *et al.*, 2002). The authors of this study commented on the awkward paradox that making the emergency contraceptive pill more easily available for women to prevent pregnancy could in fact be encouraging unsafe sexual practices.

Probably more crucial is that for most people the role of sex in their everyday lives is not primarily a health concern. Thorogood (1992) argues that sex is more likely to be informed by discourses of pleasure, risk, danger and penetration, and that while these experiences remain unacknowledged sexual health promotion is unlikely to be effective.

This is true of the gay community, where the culture of safer sex that emerged in the wake of the first AIDS crisis has now melted away (Hari, 2005). It is reported that nearly 60 per cent of gay British men had unprotected anal sex in the last year.

Part of this seemingly cavalier attitude to safer sex lies with the belief of some gay men that contracting HIV is a minor inconvenience that can be treated effectively, leading some HIV experts to label the new treatments 'protease dis-inhibitors' (DH, 2001; Hari, 2005). Again managing these perceptions is crucial if sexual health promotion is to be successful.

ISSUES OF TRUST AND POWER

Vital to any discussion on sexual health promotion is the complexity of sexual relationships and issues of power and trust within those relationships. Aggleton and Tryrer (1994) argue that for health promotion to be effective it is necessary to address the wider issues of oppression, gender inequalities, distribution of power and cultural expectations. Discussion has already alluded to the fact that sexual health decisions normally involve more than one person. Often individuals do not freely make choices about their own sexual health, for example over condom use. This is particularly true of young women's difficulties in negotiating safer sex, in which the partner's preference of method is important. Holland *et al.* (1990) found that young women often had a negative view of condoms as a form of contraception, as they were unacceptable to their current partners, while using the contraceptive pill became a symbol of their 'love and trust' for their partners. At the other end of the lifespan, older heterosexual couples often resist listening to safer sexual messages, as this would challenge the love and trust within their relationships.

DIFFICULTIES IN GETTING SEXUAL HEALTH MESSAGES ACROSS

It is often difficult to target health messages to specific groups, as individuals have different attitudes to their own sexual health, which are influenced by their own needs, self-esteem and peer norms (Mussen *et al.*, 1998). This is complicated still further in that sexual health behaviour does not occur in isolation, but involves at least one other person, and such a person may have differing sets of needs and values.

MIXED MESSAGES

This is particularly an issue for teenagers, where the adult world bombards teenagers with sexually explicit messages that give the impression that sexual activity is the norm. At the same time, the reaction of many 'adults', including parents and public institutions, to teenage sex is one of embarrassment or (worse) silence, in a mistaken belief that if sex is not talked about it won't happen. The result, for the Social Exclusion Unit (1999): 'is not less sex, but less protected sex'.

CONCLUSIONS

Sexual health is an important public health concern both nationally and internationally, and one that has been identified by the current British Government as a key policy issue. Health professionals working in the sexual health field have a vital role to play in helping to improve the sexual health of both populations and individual clients.

To achieve this professionals working in sexual health need to develop a clear understanding of their roles and responsibilities, and the relevant skills needed to undertake this work. Crucial to this understanding is the need for professionals to be cognizant of the complexity of sexual health relationships and the challenges involved in working in this difficult area of work.

REFERENCES

Abraham C, Sheeran P (1993) In search of a psychology of safer sex promotion: beyond beliefs and texts. *Health Education Research* 8(2) 245–54

Aggleton P, Tryrer P (1994) Sexual Health in Aggleton P, Rivers K, Warwick I, Whitty G (eds), *Learning About Aids: Scientific and Social Issues*, 2nd end. Churchill Livingstone/HEA, London

Alder M (2003) Sexual health: report finds services to be in a shambles. *British Medical Journal* 327 (12) 62–3

Cooper Y (2001) Foreword *Better Prevention, Better Services, Better Sexual Health: The National Strategy for Sexual Health and HIV*. Department of Health, London

DH (Department of Health) (2001) *Better Prevention, Better Services, Better Sexual Health: The National Strategy for Sexual Health and HIV*. Department of Health, London

DH (Department of Health) (2002) *The National Strategy for Sexual Health and HIV Implementation Action Plan*. Department of Health, London

DH (Department of Health) (2004a) *Choosing Health: Making Healthier Choices Easier Choices*. Department of Health, London

DH (Department of Health) (2004b) *The National Chlamydia Screening Programme in England*. Department of Health, London

DH (Department of Health) (2005) *Recommended Standards for Sexual Health Services*. Department of Health, London

Duffin A (2005) Sexual Health and Sexually Transmissible Infections in Gilly Andrews (ed.), *Women's Sexual Health*, 3rd edn. Elsevier, London

Dupont S, Webber J, Dass K, Thonton S (2002) Emergency contraceptive pill and sexual risk behaviour. *International Journal of STD and AIDS* Vol. 13, (July 2002) 482–5

Elford J, Hart G, Sherr L, Williamson L, Bolding G (2002) Peer-led HIV prevention among homosexual men in Britain. *Sexually Transmitted Infections* Vol. 78(3) (June 2002) 158–9

Ewles L, Simnet I (2003) *Promoting Health: A Practical Guide*, 5th edn. Baillière Tindall, London

Hari J (2005) Death Wish. *The Independent* Monday 7 November 2005 38–9

Hart GJ, Duncan B, Fenton KA (2002) Chlamydia Screening and Sexual Health. *Sexually Transmitted Infections* Vol. 78(6) (December 2002) 396–7

HEA (Health Education Authority) (1994) *Health Update No. 4 Sexual Health*. HEA, London

Holland J, Ramazanoglu S, Scott S (1990) Sex, Risk and Danger: Aids Education Policy and Young Women's Sexuality (WRAP Paper 1). Tufnell Press, London

HPA (Health Protection Agency) (2005) *Sexually Transmitted Infections, Epidemiological Data.* Available from: http://www.hpa.org.uk/infections/topics_az/hiv_and_sti/epidemiology/sti_data.htm Accessed 7.11.2005

Imrie J, Mercer C, Hart G, Stephenson J (2005) Move to positive prevention than sexually transmitted infection screening. *AIDS, Official Journal of the International AIDS Society* October 2005, 1708–9

Ingram Fogel, CI (1990) *Sexual Health Promotion.* W. B. Saunders, Philadelphia

McEwan R, Bhopal, R (1991) *HIV/Aids health promotion for young people: a review of the theory, principles and practice.* Health Education Authority, London

Mussen J, Naidoo J, Wills J (1998) Sexual Health Promotion in *Practising Health Promotion.* Baillière Tindall, London

Naidoo J, Wills J (1998) *Practising Health Promotion.* Baillière Tindall, London

Naidoo J, Wills J (2000) *Health Promotion: Foundations for Practice,* 2nd ed. Ballière Tindall, London

Rhodes T (1990) HIV outreach, peer education and community change: developments and dilemmas. *Health Education Journal* 53 92–9

Rooney M. Scott P (1992) Working where the risks are: health promotion interventions for men who have sex with men. In Evans B, Sandberg S, Watson S (eds), *Working Where the Risks Are: Issues in HIV Prevention.* Health Education Authority, London

Seedhouse D (2004) *Health Promotion, Philosophy, Prejudice and Practice.* Chichester, Wiley and Sons Ltd

Social Exclusion Unit (1999) *Teenage Pregnancy.* Social Exclusion Unit, London

Social Trends 33 (2003) Office of National Statistics, London

Tannahill A (1985) What is health promotion? *Health Education Journal* 44(4) 167–8

Thorogood N (1992) What is the relevance of sociology for Health Promotion? In Bunton R, MacDonald G (eds), *Health Promotion: Disciplines and Diversity.* London, Routledge

Tones K (1990) Why theorise: ideology in health education. *Health Education Journal* 49 2–6

Watney S (1990) Safer Sex as Community Practice in Aggleton P, Davies P, Hart G (eds), *Aids: Individual, Cultural and Policy Dimensions.* Falmer Press, Lewes

WHO (1946) *Constitution.* WHO, Geneva

WHO (1984) *Health Promotion: A Discussion Document on the Concept and Principles.* World Health Organisation, Copenhagen

WHO (1995) *Sexually Transmitted Diseases: Three Hundred and Thirty-Three Million New Curable Cases in 1995.* Press release WHO/64. WHO, Geneva

WHO (2002) (Internet) Gender and Reproductive Rights, Working Definitions, available from: http://www.who.int/reproductive-health/gender/sexual_health.html (accessed 07.11.2005)

10 Women's Sexual Health

GRAINNE COONEY

INTRODUCTION

The changing face of sexual health can at times make it difficult to keep up with consumer demand. In recent years a rapid increase in the number of clients of varying sexes, ages and needs attending clinic has been widely reported and accepted. This in turn has brought with it the need to adapt constantly to this growing flux of people.

The Sexual Health Strategy (DH, 2001) acknowledges that sexual health is an important part of physical and mental health. Its model states that the essential elements of good sexual health include access to information and services to avoid the risk of unintended pregnancy, illness or disease – quite a broad and complex prerequisite, I feel. However, for nurses in the field of sexual health it brings with it an equally varied array of exciting challenges to be met with on a regular basis.

This chapter will look at women-focused presentations within the sexual health setting and cover the following topics: the menstrual cycle, vaginal discharge, pelvic pain, irregular bleeding patterns, vulval pain syndromes, cervical cytology, endometriosis and fibroids.

THE MENSTRUAL CYCLE

It has been said that the human female reproductive cycle is one of the most elegant examples of endocrinology in the animal kingdom. We do not have a breeding season and, with some other higher-order primates, are the only animals that menstruate.

Historically, and for women as hunter-gathers, menarche occurred later and menopause earlier. It was also normal for lactation to continue for three to four years. As a result, women would have five to six children. Consequently, because of protracted amenorrhagia, women would experience only thirty menstruations in their lifetimes.

This is a very different picture to that of the woman of today, who will experience 450 menstruations in a lifetime. Thus in evolutionary terms repeated

Advanced Clinical Skills for GU Nurses. Edited by Matthew Grundy-Bowers and Jonathan Davies
© 2007 John Wiley & Sons Ltd

exposure to menstruation is relatively recent. With this new-found biological state, however, come new health problems.

THE MENSTRUAL CYCLE AND ITS HORMONE CONTROL

While the length of the normal menstrual cycle varies from woman to woman, the average cycle lasts 28 days. With significant variations, cycles can be as short as 21 days or as long as 36 days. Longer cycles are more common in women at the beginning or the end of their reproductive lives. This reflects the development or the deterioration, of ovarian function (Silverton, 1993).

The menstrual cycle is under the control of the higher centres of the brain (the cerebrum). It has been said that, as these areas are also concerned with the emotions, psychological upset can therefore alter menstrual regularity.

The major hormones involved in the control of reproductive function (Lewis and Chamberlain, 1990):

- *Gonadotrophin-releasing hormone (GnRH)* is a small polypeptide produced and released by the hypothalamus in pulses. It then flows through the pituitary portal system to stimulate the secretion of *luteinising hormone* (LH) and *follicle-stimulating hormone* (FSH) from the pituitary gland.
- The pulsatile secretion of *GnRH* every 90 minutes is vital for the reproductive cycle to continue. Continuous secretion of the hormone leads to decreased stimulation of the pituitary gland. The secretion of GnRH is controlled by neurotransmitters from the higher cerebral centres, and by feedback of oestrogen and progesterone from the ovary.
- *Luteinising hormone (LH) and Follicle stimulating hormone (FSH)* are two glycoproteins secreted by the pituitary in response to pulsatile GnRH, and therefore have pulsatile patterns of secretion themselves. FSH stimulates the development of Graafian follicles within the ovary.
- *Oestrogen* is secreted by the granulose and theca cells of the ovarian follicles and, after luteinisation, by the same cells in the corpus luteum. Its physiological actions include:
  Control of the monthly proliferative phase of the endometrium, with menstruation occurring following its withdrawal.
  An increase in circulating oestrogen mid-cycle that stimulates cervical glands to produce clear alkaline mucus that protects spermatozoa from the vagina's acid environment.
  Inhibition of pituitary activity through positive feedback. A rise in oestrogen concentration mid-cycle increases the sensitivity of the pituitary gonadotrophs to GnRH, increasing the frequency and height of LH pulses, and thereby increasing the LH and accompanying FSH surges that cause ovulation.

- *Progesterone* is produced by the corpus luteum. Its actions include:
  Responsibility for the luteal phase of the menstrual cycle, which will, however, only be taken up if the endometrium has already been primed by the action of oestrogens.

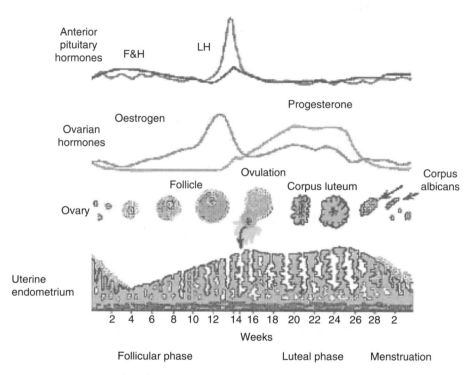

The menstrual cycle. (Reproduced by permission of the University of Wisconsin Digital Collections Center.)

The ovarian cycle describes the events that occur in the ovary during a menstrual cycle before, during and after ovulation. The ovarian cycle is divided into the follicular phase (pre-ovulatory) and the luteal phase (post-ovulatory).

THE FOLLICULAR PHASE

FSH starts to rise two days prior to menstruation, stimulating the growth and maturation of ovarian follicles. Each of these follicles consists of a maturing ovum, with surrounding granulosa and theca interna cells that are derived from the ovarian stroma. These granulosa and theca cells produce oestrogens (mainly oestradiol).

The level of *LH* is fairly constant during the follicular phase of the cycle. However, the rising *oestrogen* levels (along with increasing levels of inhibin, a polypeptide) inhibit the output of *FSH* by negative feedback, as they alter the sensitivity of the pituitary to *GnRH*. This results in a fall in FSH level on about day 5 of the menstrual cycle.

Oestrogen levels rise with continuing maturation and growth of the dominant follicle. During the final maturation phase, a rapid increase in the levels of oestrogen (around day 12) increases the sensitivity of the pituitary gonadotrophs to GnRH, in turn increasing the frequency and height of LH pulses, hence also producing the mid-cycle LH and accompanying FSH surges that cause ovulation at around day 14 (positive feedback to oestrogen). While there are up to 50 follicles beginning to mature in the early part of each cycle, generally only one matures fully and ovulates.

THE LUTEAL PHASE

When the ovum has been released from the follicle there is a temporary fall in the oestrogen level, and the FSH and LH levels are reduced. The granulosa and the theca cell of the now empty follicle become swollen and take up fat. It becomes yellow, and is thus named corpus luteum 'yellow body'. The corpus luteum secretes increasing amounts of progesterone and oestradiol, so that levels begin to rise once more.

However, *progesterone* dominates this phase. It prepares the endometrium to receive the fertilized egg if fertilisation occurs. Progesterone also alters the pituitary sensitivity to GnRH, resulting in less frequent pulses of LH, but increasing the height of each LH pulse.

If the ovum is not fertilized, there is atresia of the courpus luteum in the last week of the cycle. This results in a hyaline body known as a corpus albicans 'white body'. The levels of oestrogen and progesterone decrease, and the ovarian cycle ends as the support given to the endometrium by these hormones ceases, and menstruation occurs.

ENDOMETRIAL CYCLE

The endomctrium undergoes cyclical regeneration and disintegration under the influence of oestrogen and progesterone. The endometrium is composed of glands supported on a bed of stroma that contains fibroblasts and white blood cells. The cycle is divided into three phases.

The *menstrual phase* lasts about 4–6 days, and occurs as a result of the degeneration of the luteum following a fall in oestrogen and progesterone production. The spiral arterioles that supply the endometrium undergo vasospasm, which leads to necrosis and desquamation of the endometrium. This leaves the basal layer from which the next cycle's endometrium will form.

The proliferative/*follicular phase* starts with low levels of oestrogen, which stimulate the hypothalamus to produce FSH-releasing hormone, resulting in the release of FSH. This stimulates the developing Graafian follicle to produce oestrogen, which causes growth of the endometrium. Ovulation occurs at the end of this phase at about day 14.

In the *secretory/luteal phase,* the corpus luteum produces oestrogen and progesterone, causing the endometrium to thicken further, so becoming even more vascular. This produces an environment into which the fertilized ovum can implant and obtain nourishment.

If fertilization does not take place, the corpus luteum will start to degenerate as levels of progesterone drop. In response to this, the spiral arterioles supplying the endometrium undergo vasospasm, which leads to necrosis and desquamation of the endometrium. This results in menstruation.

CERVICAL MUCUS

In the early pre-ovulatory phase of the menstrual cycle the cervical mucus is thick, sticky and opaque. It forms a plug that blocks the cervical canal. Increasing concentrations of oestrogen alter the mucus, which becomes copious, thin elastic and clear. This facilitates the ascent of spermatozoa to the endometrial cavity and the upper genital tract. Following ovulation progesterone alters its state again. The secretions become viscid, scarce, sticky and opaque. This acts as a barrier to spermatozoa. Along with alterations in cervical mucus, there is a change in pH from 4 pre-ovulation, to a pH of 7–8 in the peri- and post-ovulatory part of the cycle.

VAGINAL DISCHARGE

Vaginal discharge varies dramatically during a woman's lifetime and during each phase of the menstrual cycle. These changes in the vaginal epithelium and vaginal secretion influence the defence against vaginal infection. Vaginal secretions consist of a mixture of vulval secretion, composed of secretions from sebaceous glands, transudates from Bartholin's and Skene's glands, and cervical mucus (Emens (1983) cited by Silverton (1993)). It also consists of vaginal transudate containing desquamated vaginal epithelial cells, giving it a creamy colour. The viscosity of the secretion is influenced mainly by the cervical component (Lewis and Chamberlain, 1990).

Vaginal secretions are acid, with a pH of 3.8–4.2 (Emens 1983) during the reproductive years. This is a result of high levels of lactic acid (2–3 per cent), which is produced by the action of commensal organisms (Doderlein's bacilli) on glycogen contained in desquamated vaginal epithelial cells. This level of acidity prevents the multiplication of most pathogenic organisms (Lewis and Chamberlain, 1992). As has been mentioned, the normal production of vaginal secretion varies considerably between individuals. This is important to bear in mind when differentiating between physiological and pathological discharges.

Table 8 Common causes of vaginal discharge

Physiological		
Age	Local factors	Hormones
Prepubertal	Menstruation	Hormonal contraception
Reproductive	Post partum	Cyclical hormonal changes
Post-menopausal	Malignancy	Pregnancy
	Semen	
	Personal habits and hygiene	

Pathological	
Infective discharge	Other cause of discharge
Conditions: • Bacterial vaginosis • Acute pelvic inflammatory disease • Pelvic infection post operatively • Puerperal sepsis	• Retained tampon or condom • Chemical irritation • Allergic responses • Ectropion • Endocervical polyp • Intrauterine device • Atrophic changes
Organisms: • *Candida albicans* • *Trichomonas vaginalis* • *Chlamydia trachomatis* • *Neisseria gonorrhoeae*	Less common causes • Physical trauma • Vault granulation tissue • Vesicovaginal fistula • Rectovaginal fistula • Neoplasia
Less common causes: • Human papillomavirus • Primary syphilis • *Mycoplasma genitalium* • *Ureaplasma urealyticum* • *Escherichia coli*	

Source: Adaped from Soutter 1998 and Mitchell 2004.

BACTERIAL VAGINOSIS

INCIDENCE AND AETIOLOGY

Bacterial vaginosis (BV) is the commonest cause of abnormal discharge in women of childbearing age. The incidence of BV varies from 5 per cent in a group of asymptomatic college students to 50 per cent of Ugandan women (BASHH, 2001). It occurs when there is a decreased number of lactobacilli and an overgrowth of organisms such as *Gardnerella vaginalis*, ureaplasmas, myco-plasmas, *Mobiluncus* species and anaerobes (Wisdom and Hawkins, 1997).

Bacterial vaginosis has been diagnosed more frequently in women who have sex with women (31.4 per cent) (Bailey *et al.*, 2004). It is also associated with a new sexual partner and frequent change of sexual partners (Mitchell, 2004).

Table 9

Signs	Symptoms
Thin white homogeneous discharge coating the walls of the vagina and vestibule	• Offensive fishy smelling discharge • Not associated with soreness, itching or irritation • Many women (approximately 50%) are asymptomatic

DIAGNOSIS

The isolation of *Gardnerella vaginalis* itself cannot be relied upon to diagnose bacterial vaginosis, as it can be cultured vaginally in more than 50 per cent of women. However, in research studies a high concentration of *Gardnerella vaginalis* is associated with the presence of bacterial vaginosis (McDonald *et al.*, 1997).

ISON/HAY CRITERIA (HAY *ET AL.* 1994)

This involves using a Gram-stained vaginal smear and grading the findings on microscopy.

Grade 1 (Normal):	*Lactobacillus* morphotypes predominate.
Grade 2 (Intermediate):	Mixed flora, with some lactobacilli present, but *Gardnerella* or *Mobiluncus* morphotypes also present.
Grade 3 (BV):	Predominantly *Gardnerella* and/or *Mobiluncus* morphotypes. Few or absent lactobacilli.

AMSEL CRITERIA (AMSEL *ET AL.* 1983)

At least three of the four criteria need to be present for the diagnosis to be confirmed.

1. Thin, white, homogeneous discharge
2. Clue cells on microscopy
3. pH of vaginal fluid > 4.5
4. Release of a fish odour on adding alkali (10 per cent).

NUGENT SCORE (NUGENT *ET AL.* 1991)

This is derived from estimating the relative proportions of bacterial morpho-types to gain a score between 0 and 10.

<4 is normal
4–6 is intermediate
>6 is bacterial vaginosis.

MANAGEMENT (BASHH, 2001)

Treatment for bacterial vaginosis is indicated for:

• Symptomatic women
• Women undergoing some surgical procedures
• Some pregnant women.

RECOMMENDED REGIMES

• Metronidazole 400–500 mg BD for 5–7 days
• Metronidazole 2 g immediately
• Other treatments include:
  ○ Intravaginal metronidazole gel (0.75 per cent) once daily for 5 days
  ○ Intravaginal clindamycin cream (2 per cent) once daily for 7 days
  ○ Clindamycin 300 mg bd for 7 days.

GENERAL ADVICE

Women should be advised to stop vaginal douching and/or the use of shower gel and/or antiseptic agents or shampoo in the bath in order to maintain the integrity of a healthy vaginal flora.

SEXUAL PARTNERS

Routine screening and treatment of male partners is not indicated. However, Berger *et al.* (1995) reported a high incidence of bacterial vaginosis in female partners of lesbians with BV. While no study has investigated the value of treating partners of lesbians simultaneously, this may be worth considering.

FOLLOW-UP

While a test of the cure is not indicated if the woman announces the cessation of her symptoms, it is recommended that pregnant women who are treated in order to prevent pre-term birth should repeat a test after one month, and treatment should be offered if the test is positive.

VULVO-VAGINAL CANDIDIASIS

INCIDENCE AND AETIOLOGY

The most common cause of vulvo-vaginal candidiasis is *Candida albicans*. Other non-albicans species, such as *C. glabrata*, account for less then 10 per cent of cases; but it is this group that may be more resistant to treatment (Kinghorn and Priestly, 1998).

Around 75 per cent of women will experience candidiasis at some time. It is usually related to pregnancy or follows antibiotic therapy. However, while sexual acquisition plays a small role in the aetiology of vulvo-vaginal candidiasis, the infection may be passed on by male partners, who can then act as asymptomatic reservoirs of re-infection. Male partners can also develop symptomatic balanitis (Kinghorn and Priestly, 1998). Ten to twenty per cent of women of reproductive age may harbour *Candida* species and remain asymptomatic, and, for these women, treatment is not required.

CLINICAL FEATURES (BASHH 2002; SOUTTER 1998)

Candida albicans and the non-albicans species share common symptoms.

Table 10 Clinical features (*Candida albicans* and non-*albicans* species share common symptoms)

Signs	Symptoms
Erythema	Vulval itching
Fissuring	Vulval soreness
Discharge: can be curdy, non-offensive	Vaginal discharge
Satellite lesions	Superficial dyspareunia
Oedema	External dysuria

DIAGNOSES (BASHH, 2002)

Clinical

- Signs and symptoms as above.

Microscopy

- Gram-staining; collection of vaginal discharge from the anterior fornix or lateral vaginal wall and identification of pseudohyphae/spores. From 65 per cent to 68 per cent of symptomatic cases can be detected in this manner.

- Saline microscopy; collection of vaginal discharge from the anterior fornix or lateral vaginal wall and identification of pseudohyphae. This gives 40–60 per cent detection.

Culture

- Sabouraud's media. Advised in all symptomatic cases where microscopy is inconclusive or species identification is helpful.

MANAGEMENT (BASHH, 2002)

General advice

Avoidance of local irritants such as bubble baths
Avoidance of tight-fitting synthetic clothing.

TREATMENT (BASHH, 2002)

Topical treatments

○ Clotrimazole pessary (500 mg stat/200 mg × 3 nights/100 × 6 nights)
○ Clotrimazole cream 10 per cent 5 g stat
○ Ecoazole pessary (150 mg stat/150 mg × 3 nights)

Oral treatments

○ Fluconazole 150 mg stat
○ Itraconazole 200 mg bd × 1 day

Sexual partners

There is no evidence to support treatment of asymptomatic sexual partners.

PREGNANCY

There is a higher incidence of asymptomatic *Candida* species colonisation during pregnancy (30–40 per cent). Symptomatic candidosis is also more prevalent during pregnancy. Oral therapy is contraindicated. Therefore treatment with topical azoles is recommended.

RECURRENT CANDIDOSIS (BASHH, 2002)

Definition

- Four or more episodes of symptomatic candidosis annually

Prevalence

- <5 per cent of healthy women of reproductive age

Pathogenesis

- Underlying immunodeficiency
- Corticosteroid use
- Frequent antibiotic use
- Diabetes mellitus

However, pathogenesis not fully understood.

Treatment regimes

- Fluconazole 100 mg weekly × 6/12
- Clotrimazole pessary 500 mg weekly × 6/12

PELVIC PAIN

Pain is defined by the International Association for the Study of Pain (1986) as 'an unpleasant sensory and emotional experience associated with actual or potential tissue damage, or described in terms of such damage'. The Royal College of Obstetrics and Gynaecology (2005) stipulate that acute pain reflects fresh tissue damage and resolves as the tissue heals. In chronic pain, additional factors are involved, and pain may continue long after the original tissue injury, or may exist in the absence of any such injury.

CAUSES OF PELVIC PAIN

Table 11 Cause of pelvic pain

Common cause of pelvic pain	
Acute	Chronic
Gynaecological	**Gynaecological**
• Infection	• Pelvic Inflammatory Disease
• Endometriosis	• Endometriosis
• Ectopic pregnancy	• Adhesions
• Cyst (bleeding or torsion)	• Fibroids
• Torsion of a fibroid	• Ovarian cyst
• Dysmenorrhoea	• Venous congestion
Non-gynaecological	**Non-gynaecological**
• Cystitis	• Irritable bowel disease
• Appendicitis	• Muscular – skeletal
• Colitis	• Bowel – urinary neoplasm
• Neurological	• Neurological
• Psychological	• Psychological

Source: Thomas and Rock 1997.

Assessment

Adequate time should be given for the initial assessment of women with pelvic pain, especially chronic pain. It has been shown that consultations that allow women to express their own ideas about their pain result in a better practitioner–patient (or therapeutic?) relationship, and therefore improved concordance with investigation and treatment (Selfe *et al.*, 1998).

History

The initial history should include questions regarding the pattern of the pain, the onset, timing, severity and type of pain, its association with other problems involving the bladder or bowel, the effect of movement and posture on pain, and the extent and type of psychological involvement. If dyspareunia occurs, is it superficial or deep, and does it occur every time? Consider also recent infection or surgery. Does the pain bear any relationship to the menstrual cycle?

Examination

Examination in a Genito-urinary Clinic should include:

- Pregnancy test
- Abdominal examination
- Perianal and vaginal speculum examination
- Sample taking for sexually and non-sexually transmitted infections
- Bimanual examination.

It is worth noting that the examiner should be prepared for new information to be revealed at this point, as the woman may now have more time/opportunity to explore her fears and anxieties.

MANAGEMENT OF PELVIC PAIN

Ectopic pregnancy

Generally there is an acute onset of symptoms. The most significant symptoms include; unilateral pelvic pain, amenorrhoea, and vaginal bleeding. The most significant signs are lower abdominal tenderness, extreme tenderness in the lateral fornix on one side, and pain on moving the cervix. Pregnancy test – Positive.

This is more common in women who have had:

- A previous ectopic pregnancy
- Tubal surgery
- Previous PID

- Tubal pathology – PID, endometriosis
- IUCD failure
- Progestogen-only methods of contraception

Urgent referral to gynaecology is imperative, as the condition may quickly become life-threatening.

Miscarriage

Spontaneous miscarriage is the expulsion of a fetus before 24 weeks. History should establish details of the last menstrual period, bleeding *per vaginam*, abdominal pain, the first positive pregnancy test, and symptoms of pregnancy. If the first evidence of miscarriage is evident at vaginal speculum examination, the cervical os will appear open, and unequivocal products of conception may be evident. Any products of conception, if passed, should be sent for histology. The woman should be referred to the local gynaecology team on call, with provisions made for safe transfer as per clinic guidelines. This will be a psychologically traumatic experience for the woman, and her management must reflect this.

Ovarian cyst

Benign ovarian cysts are common, frequently asymptomatic and often resolve spontaneously. They are the fourth most prevalent gynaecological cause of hospital admission (Soutter *et al.*, 2003). Physiological cysts are simply large versions of the cysts formed in the ovary during the normal ovarian cycle. Most are asymptomatic, being found incidentally during pelvic examination. Management is conservative, though pelvic scan should be considered if the pain is moderate and there are few physical signs. If the patient presents with severe acute pain or bleeding a laparoscopy or laparotomy under the care of a gynaecology team is indicated.

PELVIC INFLAMMATORY DISEASE (PID)

As has been indicated earlier, Pelvic Inflammatory Disease may be either acute or chronic. PID is a common cause of morbidity, and accounts for 1 in 60 consultations by women under the age of 45 (Simms *et al.*, 2000). It has been reported that a delay of a few days in receiving appropriate treatment can increase the risk of sequelae, which include infertility, ectopic pregnancy and chronic pelvic pain (Hillis *et al.*, 1993).

The RCOG Guidance (2003) recommends that, owing to a lack of definitive clinical diagnostic criteria, a low threshold for the empirical treatment of

PID is recommended. They also suggest that in severe cases, or where there is diagnostic doubt, the woman should be admitted to hospital for further investigation and treatment.

CAUSES

PID is usually the result of ascending infection from the endocervix, causing endometritis, salpingitis, parametritis, oophoritis, tubo-ovarian abscess and/or pelvic peritonitis. Sexually transmitted infections, such as *Chlamydia trachomatis* and *Neisseria gonorrhoeae* are identified as causative agents. *Mycoplasma genitalium* anaerobes and other organisms may also be implicated (Bevan *et al.*, 1995).

CLINICAL FEATURES

- Lower abdominal pain and tenderness
- Deep dyspareunia
- Abnormal vaginal or cervical discharge
- Abnormal vaginal bleeding
- Cervical excitation and adnexal tenderness on motion
- Fever (>38°C)
- Nausea and vomiting

SHORT-TERM COMPLICATIONS

Fitz-Hugh–Curtis syndrome

This takes the form of peri-hepatitis and is generally chlamydial or gonococcal in origin. Laparoscopy reveals oedema of the liver capsule and adhesions to the peritoneum.

Pelvic abscess

These are detected by the palpation of an adnexal mass, confirmed by ultrasound. Antibiotics may reduce the abscess, but occasionally surgery is necessary.

LONG-TERM COMPLICATIONS

Chronic pain

The exact origin of chronic pelvic pain is difficult to ascertain. It may be due to recurrence of infection or adhesions and scarring in the pelvic cavity caused by previous infection. The patient may present with pain following sexual intercourse or with pain during a certain time in the menstrual cycle as organs move in response to hormonal influence.

Recurrence

Subsequent attacks are said to be more likely after one episode of PID.

Ectopic pregnancy

Owing to scarring in the Fallopian tubes, ectopic pregnancies are more likely in women who have earlier suffered from PID.

Impaired fertility

Again as a result of the scarring following each episode of PID, the likelihood of fertility impairment increases.

Diagnosis

Clinical symptoms and signs lack sensitivity and specificity (the positive predictive value of clinical diagnosis is 65–90 per cent compared with laparoscopic diagnosis) (Bevan *et al.*, 1995). Microbiological tests for gonorrhoea and *Chlamydia* in the lower genital tract are recommended, as a positive result strongly supports the diagnosis of PID (Bevan *et al.*, 1995; Morcos *et al.*, 1993). An elevated erythrocyte sedimentation rate (ESR) or c-reactive protein rate (CRP) also supports the diagnosis (Miettinen *et al.*, 1993). While laparoscopy may strongly support a diagnosis of PID, it is not routinely justified on the basis of cost. Endometrial biopsy and ultrasound scanning may also be helpful when there is diagnostic difficulty; but there is insufficient evidence to support their routine use at present. The absence of endocervical or vaginal pus cells has a good negative predictive value (95 per cent) for a diagnosis of PID, but their presence is non-specific (poor positive predictive value: Yudin *et al.*, 2003).

MANAGEMENT (BASHH, 2005)

Medical

Adequate pain relief is essential. BASHH guidelines (2005) recommend a low threshold for the empiric treatment of PID. Broad-spectrum antibiotics are suggested to cover gonorrhoea and *Chlamydia* along with the treatment of aerobic and anaerobic bacteria. BASHH also recommend women who are at high risk of gonococcal PID being treated with a cephalosporin-based regimen as opposed to a quinolone-based one. Overall treatment is influenced by robust evidence on local antimicrobial sensitivity patterns, the specific infection in this setting, costs, patient preferences and compliance, along with the severity of the infection.

Metronidazole is included to improve the coverage for anaerobic bacteria. Anaerobes are of relatively greater importance in patients with severe PID, and metronidazole may be discontinued in those patients with mild or moderate PID who are unable to tolerate it.

Intrauterine coil device

Faculty of Family Planning Guidelines (2004), recommend that there is no need to remove an intrauterine device unless symptoms fail to resolve.

Pregnancy and breastfeeding

- PID in pregnancy is associated with an increase in both maternal and fetal morbidity; therefore parenteral therapy is advised, although none of the suggested evidence-based regimens are of proven safety in this situation.
- There are insufficient data from clinical trials to recommend a specific regimen.
- The risk of giving any of the recommended antibiotic regimens in very early pregnancy (prior to a positive pregnancy test) is low, with any significant drug toxicity resulting in failed implantation (BASHH, 2005).

Surgical management

- Laparoscopy – division of adhesions and drainage of pelvic abscesses. Ultrasound-guided aspiration of pelvic fluid.

Follow-up

A 72-hour review is recommended for those with moderate or severe clinical presentation. If there is not substantial improvement at this point further investigation as an inpatient, parenteral therapy and/or surgical intervention may be necessary.

A four-week review following therapy will ensure:

1. an adequate clinical response to treatment;
2. compliance with oral antibiotics;
3. screening and treatment of sexual contacts; and
4. awareness of the significance of PID and its sequelae.

IRREGULAR BLEEDING PATTERNS

MENORRHAGIA

Menorrhagia is defined as a complaint of heavy cyclical menstrual bleeding over several consecutive cycles. It is also worth being aware that an average menstrual cycle occurs every 21 to 35 days and last from 2 to 7 days. Normal blood flow is 30 to 80 ml (RCOG, 2004). Menorrhagia can be defined objectively or subjectively. Objective menorrhagia is taken to be a total menstrual blood loss of 80 ml or more. Subjective menorrhagia is defined as a complaint of excessive menstrual blood loss over several consecutive cycles in a woman of reproductive years.

Epidemiology

Menorrhagia has an impact on many women's lives, with 1 in 20 women aged 30–49 consulting her GP each year with this complaint. On referral to a gynaecologist, surgical intervention is highly likely, with 1 in 5 women in the UK having a hysterectomy before the age of 60 years. About half of all women who have a hysterectomy for menorrhagia have a normal uterus removed (RCOG, 1999).

Pathogenesis

Menorrhagia is thought to be associated with uterine fibroids, adenomyosis, pelvic infection, endometrial polyps and the presence of a foreign body such as an intrauterine contraceptive device. Lumsden and Norman (1998) state that in women with menstrual blood loss greater than 200 ml, over half will have fibroids, although only 40 per cent of those with adenomyosis actually have menstrual blood loss in excess of 80 ml. According to Hurskainen et al., (1999) approximately half of the cases who present with menorrhagia show no underlying pathology. It is thought that vascular changes may play an important role, but the condition remains poorly understood.

Diagnosis and management of menorrhagia (See Table 12)

Treatment should take into consideration patients' issues. Women should be included in the decision-making process. Surgical treatment should only be carried out with outcomes and complications explained. Quality of life issues should be addressed.

Table 12

History (A full gynaecological history should be taken)	Heavy cyclical menstrual blood loss over several consecutive cycles without any intermenstrual or post-coital bleeding (RCOG 1998)	*Note*: Symptoms of other pathology include: • Irregular bleeding • Sudden change in blood loss • Intermenstrual bleeding • Postcoital bleeding • Dyspareunia • Pelvic pain • Premenstrual pain *Risk factors for oestrogen treatments*: • Polycystic Ovary Syndrome • Obesity (RCOG 1998)
Examination	Bimanual abdominal examination • Cervical smear if due • Sexual health screen if history suggests pregnancy test	*Note*: • If uterus enlarged, i.e. above 10 weeks in size, if there is pelvic masses or tenderness noted, refer appropriately. • If pregnancy test positive, refer appropriately
Investigation	Full blood count	*Note*: Treat for anaemia if anaemic

Amended from: Royal College of Obstetrics and Gunaerology, 1998.

Drug treatment

Second-line drugs include danazole and gonadotrophin-releasing hormone analogues which are shown to be effective in reducing heavy menstrual blood loss, but side-effects limit their long-term use. Progestogen-releasing intrauterine systems reduce heavy menstrual blood loss and are a good alternative to surgical treatment.

Surgical treatments

- Hysteroscopic removal of submucous fibroids or polyps.
- Endometrial ablative procedures are effective in treating menorrhagia.
- Hysterectomy – should be balanced against its potential mortality and morbidity.

(RCOG, 2004)

DYSFUNCTIONAL UTERINE BLEEDING

The term 'dysfunctional uterine bleeding' refers to those cases in which the bleeding is not due to some diagnosed local disorder, such as new growth or pelvic infection, or some complication of pregnancy. It may occur at any age between menarche and menopause (Lewis and Chamberlain, 1990). Lewis and Chamberlain (2004) go on to explain that heavy or irregular bleeding without abnormal physical signs on ordinary examination will always suggest this diagnosis, but must never be taken for granted, as curettage may reveal that there is a local cause for the bleeding after all.

PATHOGENESIS

The causes of dysfunctional uterine bleeding appears to be mainly hormonal in origin. The abnormalities of ovarian activity may be classed as 'ovulatory' or 'anovulatory' (Lumsden and Norman, 1998).

In *anovulatory cycles*, which can occur for all women, normal amounts of oestrogen are secreted, but the egg may not ripen in the follicle. As an egg is not released, progesterone is not produced from the corpus luteum to counteract the proliferation of the uterine lining. In time the uterine lining outgrows its blood supply, and sloughs off at irregular intervals. Anovulation may be a result of inadequate signals, for example as a result of polycystic ovarian disease, or it may be pre-menopausal. It may also be caused by impaired positive feedback, for example in adolescence.

Ovulatory causes may result from an inadequate luteal phase that occurs if there is an insufficient peak in progesterone. This is usually a result of a reduced amount of follicle-stimulating hormone being secreted. This syndrome may be associated with irregular bleeding and infertility.

Another area that may cause dysfunctional bleeding is at the site of vasoconstriction, where the bleeding is caused by an imbalance of vasoconstrictor prostaglandins and vasodilator prostaglandins. The cause for this is still under review.

DIAGNOSIS AND MANAGEMENT

As per menorrhagia.

INTERMENSTRUAL BLEEDING

Intermenstrual bleeding is defined as any bleeding occurring within a regular menstrual cycle but not at menstruation.

PATHOGENESIS

- Infection
- Physiological (see below for more detail)
- Cervical erosion (see below for more detail)

- Oral contraceptive (see below for more detail)
- Vulvitis
- Cervical cell abnormality

INVESTIGATION

A complete history should be taken, along with a sexual health screen and examination. If indicated, a cervical smear should be performed.

MANAGEMENT

Investigate for infection. Examination to reveal masses or lesions. Consider cytology: past results/need to repeat cytology. Any abnormalities should be referred on for specialist review, as should recurring symptoms without obvious pathology. Every case of intermenstrual bleeding at any age should have a diagnosis established before treatment is given, otherwise an occasional carcinoma may be missed, sometimes with fatal results.

POST-COITAL BLEEDING

Post-coital bleeding is any bleeding occurring after intercourse.

PATHOGENESIS

- Infection
- Physiological (see below for more detail)
- Cervical erosion (see below for more detail)
- Oral contraceptive (see below for more detail)
- Vulvitis
- Cervical cell abnormality

INVESTIGATION

A complete history should be taken, along with a sexual health screen and examination. If indicated, a cervical smear should be performed.

MANAGEMENT

As per intermenstrual bleeding.

POSTMENOPAUSAL BLEEDING

Postmenopausal bleeding is defined as an episode of vaginal bleeding occurring more than 1 year after the presumed menopause.

PATHOGENESIS

- Atrophic vaginitis
- Cervical carcinoma
- Carcinoma of the endometrium

INVESTIGATION

A complete history should be taken along with a sexual health screen and examination. If indicated, a cervical smear should be performed.

MANAGEMENT

Postmenopausal bleeding should be referred to a gynaecologist after investigations for infection, and a cervical smear conducted if indicated.

MORE COMMON CAUSES OF IRREGULAR BLEEDING IN GREATER DETAIL

PHYSIOLOGICAL

Serum concentration of oestrogen fluctuates during a normal menstrual cycle. There is a large rise during the follicular phase, followed by a precipitate fall for 2 to 3 days at the time of ovulation. In some women, this fall can be so great that the endometrium loses its hormonal support in the same way as at menstruation. Desquamation commences, but stops when oestrogen and progesterone from the corpus luteum stimulate the endometrium. This is one reason why consistent mid-cycle intermenstrual bleeding is a normal phenomenon in some young women.

CERVICAL EROSION

The cervix is composed of two types of epithelium. Columnar epithelium is generally inside the cervical canal, and therefore not seen. This epithelial cell is translucent, and therefore underlying blood vessels are visible if they migrate to the extracervical area. Squamous epithelium covers the intravaginal portion of the cervix, and is generally seen. Its appearance is opaque and dull to the eye. Where the two types of epithelium meet is the squamo–columnar junction (S–C J). This junction moves up and down the cervix as the epithelia change from one type to another. These changes occur during exposure to high oestrogen levels, for example at puberty, during the use of oral contraceptives, and during pregnancy. An eversion occurs when the S–C J moves down the cervix.

The main problems caused by the columnar epithelium becoming intravaginal are that it can increase vaginal discharge, or, because the epithelium is fragile, it can become traumatised during intercourse and bleed. Eversions do not require treatment unless a cervical smear is abnormal. However, some women may require symptomatic relief with treatments such as cryotherapy or cautery.

ORAL CONTRACEPTIVES

The combined oral contraceptive pill maintains the integrity of the endometrium during the three weeks for which it is taken. Some women may have a pharmacodynamic reason as to why they do not absorb a particular oestrogen or progestogen efficiently, or their endometrium may not respond adequately to those compounds. If this is so, the endometrium will shed and the woman will experience intermenstrual bleeding. This is common during the first few months of starting a new pill. If it does not resolve it is worth considering changing to a pill with different doses of progestogen and oestrogen. It is also worthwhile considering sexual health screening and cervical cytology, to rule out any possible underlying pathology.

VULVAL PAIN SYNDROMES

VULVODYNIA

It appears that as the classification and terminology of vulvodynia evolves it may be becoming more perplexing for many health professionals to comprehend. Typically, 'vulvodynia' is a term used to describe chronic burning and/or pain in the vulva without objective physical findings to explain the symptoms (Lotery *et al.*, 2004). Within the spectrum of vulvodynia, there are several subsets. The two main ones are vulval vestibulitis and dyaesthetic vulvodynia. Others described by Julius and Metts (1999) include: papulosquamous vulvar dermatoses, vesiculobullous vulvar dermatoses, neoplastic vulvar lesions, and vestibular papillomatosis.

Lotery *et al.* (2004), advise that there are many common conditions which may cause vulval burning and/or pain, and recommend that these are excluded when evaluating chronic vulval symptoms. These include:

Irritant dermatitis, caused by irritants such as: soap, panty-liners, moistened wipes, douches, lubricants, or excessive vaginal discharge.
Candidiasis can cause vulval burning, and its treatment has been reported to improve symptoms.
Other causes include: vulvo-vaginal atrophy, recurrent *Herpes simplex* infection, *Herpes zoster* and post–herpetic neuralgia, lichen sclerosus, Behçet's syndrome, and vulval intraepithelial neoplasia.

To date, while it cannot be said that there is no specific cause underlying the burning in these patients, it would be reasonable to suggest that we are unable to determine what it is (Kaufman *et al.*, 1994 cited by Lotery *et al.*, 2004).

Historically, there have been some links made between vulvodynia and sexual and physical abuse. Most relevant studies have failed to demonstrate this link (Edwards *et al.*, 1997). Studies in which patients have more depressive symptoms and somatic complaints than controls do not differentiate between cause and effect (Lotery *et al.*, 2004). James Aikens *et al.* (2003) showed that increased scores for somatic depressive symptoms were due to a lack of sexual interest and chronic pain, with no significant difference in cognitive affective symptoms or depressive history disorder.

Epidemiology

There are few data on the incidence and prevalence of vulvodynia. The age-range seems to lie between 20 and 60 years, and it appears to be limited almost exclusively to Caucasian women. Risk-taking sexual behaviour and a history of sexually transmitted diseases are rare. Obstetric and gynaecological history is usually unexceptional (Julius and Metts, 1999).

Initial history to determine possible cause

1. Elicit exact symptoms and location of symptoms, any previous diagnosis and treatments, use of skin irritants.
2. *Examination of skin*: If there is an obvious abnormality swab for microscopy and culture, and consider a skin biopsy. If a diagnosis is made, treat accordingly. It is suggested that vaginal swabs should be taken routinely for microscopy and cultures to rule out yeast, bacterial infections, etc. (Lotery *et al.*, 2004).

DYSAESTHETIC VULVODYNIA

Dysaesthetic vulvodynia is a diagnosis given to cases of unprovoked vulval burning not limited to the vestibule and with no demonstrable abnormalities (McKay, 1988). It is mainly described in older women, who have burning that extends beyond the vaginal introitus to involve the labia majora and occasionally the inner thighs and anus. Uncontrolled observations have made links between diffuse vulval pain with low back pain or trauma, *Herpes simplex* virus, and pelvic surgery, which some investigators describe as pudendal neuralgia (McKay, 1993; Turner and Marinoff, 1991). However, there has been no data to support pudendal nerve dysfunction as a cause of vulval pain (Lotery *et al.*, 2004).

Table 13 Management of dyaesthetic vulvodynia

Typical history	Physical findings	Suggested treatment
• Usually postmenopausal or perimenopausal • Diffuse, unremitting burning pain that is not cyclic and can be unprovoked • Less dyspareunia or point tenderness than in vulvar vestibulitis	• Usually no erythematous cutaneous changes	• Tricyclic antidepressants • Gabapentin • ?consider other therapies, e.g. acupuncture (Lotery *et al.* 2004) • Counselling and support

Adapted from: Julius & Metts 1999 and Lotery *et al.* 2004.

VULVAL VESTIBULITIS (VESTIBULITIS)

Vulvar vestibulitis is typified by painful areas on the skin of the vestibules. In 1987 Friedrich set out a diagnostic criterion for vulval vestibulitis:

• Severe pain on vestibular touch or attempted vaginal entry
• Tenderness to pressure localised within the vulvar vestibule when touched with a swab
• Physical findings of erythema limited to the vulvar vestibule

It is worth bearing in mind that the vestibular area of the vagina covers many parts, including:

• Bartholin's glands
• Urethra
• Vestibular glands

PATHOGENESIS

In papers by Lotery *et al.* (2004) and Green *et al.* (2001) several causes for vestibulitis are debated. These include the absence or presence of inflammation in the vestibular tissue, and infections such as *Candida* and human papillomavirus, family history and contact dermatitis. They advise that there are no studies to substantiate these. An abnormal pain syndrome or an immunological role in the causation of vestibulitis are also discussed; but again Lotery *et al.* (2004) and Green *et al.* (2001) conclude that there is little evidence at present to sustain these causes.

Table 14 Management of vulval vestibulitis

Typical history	Physical findings	Suggested treatment
• Usually premenopausal • Entry dyspareunia or pain with insertion of tampon or intercourse • Severe pain with pressure • Burning stinging irritation or raw sensation within vestibular area • Possible history of carbon dioxide laser therapy, cryotherapy, allergic drug reactions or recent use of chemical irritants	• Positive swab test (vestibular point tenderness when touched with cotton swab) • Focal or diffuse vestibular erythema	• 5% lignocaine ointment • Tricyclic antidepressants • Gabapentin • Pelvic floor physiotherapy • ?consider local interferon injection • ?consider surgery (Lotery *et al.* 2004) • Counselling and support

Adapted from: Julius & Metts 1999 and Lotery *et al.* 2004.

CERVICAL SMEARS

Cervical screening is not a test for cancer. It is a method of preventing cancer by detecting and treating early abnormalities that, if left untreated, could lead to cervical cancer. The National Screening Programme came about following *Health of the Nation* (DH, 1993). Since its implementation, the NHS Cervical Screening Programme has been remarkably successful. It has saved a large number of women's lives and will continue to prevent about 4,500 deaths every year in England.

ELIGIBILITY

All women between the ages of 25 and 64 are eligible for a free cervical smear test every three or five years.

Reasons why women under 25 and women over 65 are not invited for cervical cytology (Sasieni *et al.*, 2003):

- Invasive cancer in women under 25 is rare, but changes in the cervix are common. This may mean that younger women may get an abnormal result when there is nothing wrong.
- Evidence suggests that screening women under the age of 25 may do more harm than good by resulting in unnecessary investigations after false positive results. It is suggested that screening women from the age of 25 will help reduce anxiety as well as the number of unnecessary investigations and treatments in younger women.
- Women aged 65 and over who have had three consecutive negative cervical tests in the preceding ten years are taken out of the recall system. The natural history and progression of cervical cancer means it is highly unlikely that such women will go on to develop the disease.
- Women aged 65 and over who have never had a screen are entitled to one.

The NHS call and recall system invites women to attend their local GP for a screen. Women must be advised to register with a local GP clinic.

RISK FACTORS FOR CERVICAL CANCER

- Certain types of human papilloma virus (HPV) are linked with around 95 per cent of all cases of cervical cancer (mainly types 16, 18, 31, and 33).
- Women with many sexual partners or whose partners have many partners.
- Long-term use of oral contraceptives increases the risk (taking the combined oral contraceptive for 5 years or more in the presence of HPV virus). Condom use gives some protection.
- Women who smoke are twice as likely to develop cancer as non-smokers.
- Women with late first pregnancy have a lower risk than those with an early pregnancy; the risk increases with the number of pregnancies.
- Women in manual social classes are more at risk than those in a non-manual social class.

Assessment of the cervix

The cervix is composed of two types of epithelium.

Columnar epithelium is generally inside the cervical canal, and therefore not usually seen. It is translucent and blood vessels are visible.
Squamous epithelium covers the intravaginal portion of the cervix. Its appearance is opaque and dull to the eye.

Where the different epithelia meet is the squamo–columnar junction (S–C J). This exposed area of columnar epithelium on the ectocervix, over a number of years, is replaced by squamous epithelium by a process of metaplasia. This area is known as the transformation zone. It is this part of the transformation zone that is adjacent to the squamo–columnar junction that is most vulnerable to cervical intraepithelial neoplasia. Therefore, when the squamo–columnar junction is visible, the cervical sample must include the whole circumference of the S–C J and the adjacent 1 cm of squamous epithelium.

As has been mentioned, columnar epithelium appears red to the eye. While this is sometimes referred to as an 'angry' cervix, 'erosion' (though the surface is not eroded), or 'ectopy' (though the columnar junction is not ectopic or misplaced) a more accurate term is **eversion**. Laceration of the cervix associated with childbirth (**ectropion**) may expose more of the canal lined by columnar epithelium. This may be further exaggerated by opening the speculum. **Nabothian follicles** may also be seen on the cervix. As a result the cervix may have a knobbly appearance. These are mucus-retaining cysts caused by normal changes of surface columnar squamous epithelium. They are generally around 5 mm in diameter, but may be enlarged to 1 to 1.5 cm. **Polyps** may be seen on the cervix. Most are entirely benign and give rise to no symptoms.

Clinical suspicion of malignancy may include: an enlarged cervix with an irregular friable surface that is crumbling to the touch, large blood vessels that may bleed freely when rubbed by the end of the speculum, and sweet smelling but offensive watery discharge (NHSCSP, 1998).

METHODS OF SCREENING

The first stage in cervical screening is either a smear test or liquid-based cytology (LBC).

Smear test (traditional)

A smear test involves a sample of cells that have been taken from the transformation zone (TZ) of the cervix for analysis. This is done by speculum examination: a spatula is used to sweep around the TZ; if the TZ is not visible, a cervical brush should be used as well.

Liquid-based cytology

Liquid-based cytology (LBC) is a technology whereby a cervix brush sample is suspended in buffer and processed so that a thin layer of cells is produced on a slide without contamination by blood cells and debris. This results in preparations that are generally easier to read. Its advantage is in a reduction in inadequate samples from 9 per cent to 1–2 per cent, and there may be gains in reducing borderline results and increasing sensitivity.

RESULTS AND TREATMENT FOLLLOWING CERVICAL SMEAR

Table 15

Grade	Explanation	Action
Negative	No abnormalities detected	Routine recall after three to five years
Abnormal	Cellular appearances which cannot be described as normal	Refer for colposcopy after one borderline change or three abnormal tests at any grade in a ten-year period
Borderline changes	Endocervical cell changes Squamous cell changes	Refer for colposcopy after one test is reported as borderline. Refer for colposcopy after three tests in a series are reported as borderline.
Mild dyskaryosis	Cellular appearances consistent with CIN 1	Ideally refer for colposcopy, but it remains acceptable to recommend a repeat test after one test reported as mild dyskaryosis. If two tests are reported as mild dysdaryosis refer for colposcopy.
Moderate dyskaryosis	Cellular appearances consistent with CIN 2	Refer for colposcopy
Severe dyskaryosis	Celluar appearances consistent with CIN 3	Refer for colposcopy
Suspected invasive cancer	Possibility of invasive cancer	Refer for colposcopy Women should be seen urgently within two weeks of referral.
Inadequate	The test cannot be interpreted. It may be too thick or too thin, obscured by inflammatory cells or blood, or incorrectly labeled; or it does not contain the right type of cell.	Repeat the best. Refer for colposcopy after three consecutive inadequate samples.

Source: NHS Publication No. 20: Colposcopy and Programme Management Guidelines for the NHS Cervical Screening Programmes.

Treatment

- There are two main methods of treatment. The abnormal cells in the cervix may be destroyed using laser ablation or cold coagulation treatments, or the abnormality may be excised using a loop diathermy or laser excision. Loop diathermy is the most common and effective treatment, and is used by 71 per cent of clinics.

- Hysterectomy is not usually necessary for CIN, as treatment aims to preserve a woman's fertility.
- Surgery is the main form of treatment for localised cases for the few women who have cancer, while radiotherapy and chemotherapy may be used for more extensive disease.

SPECIAL CONSIDERATIONS (NHSCSP (2004)):

Cervical cytology in GUM Clinics

The NHS Cervical Screening Programme (2004), suggests that cervical cytology in GUM clinics should be reserved for those with a cytological indication or those who have not been screened in previous routine screening at the appropriate interval.

Cervical screening in pregnancy

Unless a pregnant woman with a negative history has gone beyond three years without having a cervical screening then the test should be postponed. If a woman has been called for routine screening and she is pregnant then the test should be deferred. If an earlier test was abnormal, and in the interim the woman becomes pregnant, then the test should not be delayed, but should be taken in the middle trimester unless there is a clinical indication.

HIV-positive women

All women newly diagnosed with HIV should have cervical surveillance performed by, or in conjunction with, the medical team managing the HIV infection. Annual cytology may be indicated depending on disease progression, refer to local guidelines. Colposcopy for cytological abnormality should follow national/local guidelines. As there is a lack of information on the management of women from the age of 65 who are HIV-positive, it is advisable to seek local guidance in these cases.

Women who have sex with women

There is no mention of management of smears for women who have sex with women in the national screening guidelines. They do recommend that women who are not sexually active, but have had sex with men in the past, continue with the screening programme. There appears to be an overall lack of information on the cervical screening needs of women who have sex with women. It is worth noting, however, that Fethers et al. (2000) highlight no difference in the prevalence of abnormal cervical cytology and of changes suggestive of cervical intraepithelial neoplasia (CIN 1, 2, or 3) in women who have sex with women as against women who have sex with men.

ENDOMETRIOSIS

Endometriosis may be defined as a disease characterized by the presence of functioning endometrial tissue, normally situated in the uterine cavity, outside the uterus. It is most commonly found in the pelvis, but can also be present in areas such as the abdominal cavity and the pleura (Thomas and Rock, 1997).

EPIDEMIOLOGY

Endometriosis is more commonly seen in women being investigated for infertility (21%) than among those undergoing sterilization (6%). The incidence of endometriosis in women being examined for chronic abdominal pain is 15% and, for those undergoing abdominal hysterectomy, 25% (Green Top Guidelines, 2000).

AETIOLOGY AND PATHOGENESIS

Thomas and Rock (1997) indicate that factors that increase the exposure to menstruation increase the likelihood of the disease occurring, whereas those that decrease the exposure protect against it.

Aetiological factors influencing endometriosis

- Age
- Family history
- Heavy periods
- Frequent cycles
- Pregnancy protects
- Oral contraceptives protect

Menstruum not only flows down the vagina but can also reflux along the fallopian tubes and into the pelvis. It is this refluxed menstruum that is thought to be the cause of endometriosis, though the mechanism remains unknown. However, there are various suggested theories (Thomas and Rock, 1997):

Implantation

Minute fragments of endometrium pass along the fallopian tubes during menstruation and spill into the pelvic part of the peritoneal cavity; this becomes implanted on another pelvic structure such as the ovary, and develops into endometriosis. While shed endometrium is generally necrotic, living fragments have also been found.

Metaplasia of the coelomic membrane

The epithelium from the pelvis develops into endometrium-like tissue following prolonged irritation or oestrogen stimulation.

Mechanical transplantation

During surgery, endometrial tissue can be transferred from its original site to another by surgical implements such as a blade.

Vascular/Lymphatic spread

Endometrium has been found in the blood vessels and lymph channels that drain the uterus.

SIGNS AND SYMPTOMS OF ENDOMETRIOSIS

Signs

- Pelvic pain (generally cyclical)
- Dyspareunia
- Dysmenorrhoea

Symptoms

- Tender nodules on the utero-sacral ligaments
- Pelvic mass
- Pelvic fixity
- Pelvic tenderness
- Painful periods
- Heavy or irregular periods
- Diarrhoea and painful bowel movements during menstruation

DIAGNOSIS

Laparoscopy

Laparoscopy is considered the gold standard diagnostic test for endometriosis. It is, however, associated with a 0.06 per cent risk of major complications such as bowel perforation. This risk is increased to 1.3 per cent in operative laparoscopy.

Transvaginal ultrasound

The use of transvaginal ultrasound may be helpful in diagnosis, but is more so in detecting ovarian endometriomas. Magnetic resonance imaging may be a useful non-invasive tool in the diagnosis of deep endometriosis.

Serum CA-125 testing

It has been concluded that CA-125 has a limited value as a screening test as well as a diagnostic test. It may, however, serve as a useful marker for monitoring the effect of treatment following diagnosis. The Royal College of Obstetrics and Gynaecologists (RCOG, 2000) highlight the fact that its use to date has not been evaluated systematically.

MEDICAL MANAGEMENT OF ENDOMETRIOSIS AND PAIN

Non steroidal anti-inflammatory drugs

These inhibit prostaglandin synthesis and are beneficial for dysmenorrhoea. The aim of medical treatment is to induce atrophy in the ectopic endometrial tissue with the use of hormones. However, the drugs used come with some significant side-effects that limit their long-term use and often produce poor compliance. Symptom recurrence is common following medical treatment. In a follow-up study (Moore *et al.*, 1999) the cumulative recurrence rates for the fifth year after the completion of GnRH agonist treatment were 37 per cent for minimal disease and 74 per cent for severe disease.

GnRH agonists

As analogues of GnRH (gonadotropin-releasing hormone) agonists suppress LH (luteinising hormone) and FHS (follide-stimulating hormone) secretion from the pituitary. This results in ovarian suppression and significant reduction in the secretion of oestrogen, which results in thinning of the endometrium. They are generally only given for a 6-month period, as 6 per cent of bone mineral density may be lost in the first 6 months. It takes two years for the loss to be restored. It can provide up to 90 per cent relief of symptoms in patients.

Danazol

A synthetic androgen derived from 19-nortestosterone. It inhibits pituitary gonadotrophins. Similar consideration should be given to this as 60 GnRH agonists. It can provide up to 90 per cent symptom relief in patients.

Progestogens

Synthetic progestogens, medroxyprogesterone acetate and dydrogesterone are licensed for the treatment of endometriosis. They act by causing decidualisation and subsequent necrosis. While progestogens provide relief in 70–80 per cent of patients, their progestogenic side-effects (spotting, weight gain) can result in cessation of treatment.

Combined oral contraceptive pill (COC)

The therapeutic use of COC monthly or tricycling can also reduce the pain symptoms of endometriosis, as it too creates endometrial thinning and reduction in ovarian function. Tricycling can create extended periods without endometrial shedding.

Surgical management of endometriosis and pain

Laparoscopic ablation of minimal–moderate endometriosis appears to relieve pain, though it is still unclear whether uterine nerve ablation is required as well. This may also improve fertility rates.

FIBROIDS

Uterine fibroids are common benign tumours that arise from the uterine myometrium or, less commonly, from the cervix (West, 1998). The prevalence of fibroids is 20 per cent in the Caucasian population and 50 per cent in the Afro-Caribbean and Afro-American population (West, 1998).

AETIOLOGY AND PATHOGENESIS

Fibroids are derived from single myometrial cells, though G – 6 PD type may vary between individual fibroids within the same uterus (West, 1998). It is thought that fibroid growth is dependent on ovarian hormones, as they do not occur prior to menarche and normally reduce in size following menopause. Fibroids appear to develop and be maintained in response to oestrogen, and progesterone may have a major role to play in the control of fibroid growth.

CLASSIFICATION

Fibroids may be single, but are more commonly multiple and at varying sites and sizes. They are named depending on where they are located within the muscle of the uterus. They include:

• Intramural fibroids: within the muscle layer of the uterus.
• Submucosal, pedunculated submucosal or pedunculated vaginal: growing into the uterine cavity.
• Cervical subserosal, intraligamentous or pedunculated: growing outwards from the uterus.

PRESENTATION (WEST, 1998)

Menorrhagia

Between 30 and 50 per cent of women with fibroids will have menorrhagia. As menorrhagia attributable to fibroids may be very heavy, iron-deficiency anaemia may develop.

Pelvic pain and pressure

While fibroids do not always give rise to pain, their presentation may be acute on account of torsion or degeneration.

Subfertility

It is estimated that infertility is a major presenting factor or secondary feature in 27 per cent of women with fibroids.

INVESTIGATION

The most useful diagnostic tool for fibroids is pelvic ultrasound, with a full blood count and an iron study to assess anaemia. Computerised tomography (CT) scans or magnetic resonance imaging (MRI) can also be used to image fibroids, but are thought to be too expensive and show little added benefit over ultrasonography. Submucous fibroids can be found following hysterectomy.

MANAGEMENT FOLLOWING FIBROIDS SUSPECTED ON EXAMINATION

If the condition is asymptomatic – refer for an ultrasound scan. If the ultrasound scan is normal, reassure and investigate other causes. If the ultrasound is abnormal, refer to a gynaecologist.

If the condition is symptomatic – refer for an ultrasound scan and to a gynaecologist.

Table 16 Treatment of fibroids

Medical	Surgical
• Oral contraceptives	• Myomectomy
• NDAIDS	• Hysteroscpic resection
• GnRH agonists	• Hysterectomy
	• Laser ablation

Amended from: West 1998.

REFERENCES

Aikens J et al. (2003) cited in Lotery H, McClure N, Galash R (2004) Vulvodynia. *The Lancet* 363/9414 1058–61

Amsel R, Totten PA, Spiegel CA, Chen KC, Eschenbach D, Holmes KK (1983) Non-specific vaginitis. Diagnostic criteria and microbial and epidemiologic associations. *American Journal of Medicine* 74 14–22

Bailey J, Farquhar G, Owen C, Mangtani P (2004) Sexually transmitted infections in women who have sex with women. *Sexually Transmitted Infections* 80 244–6

BASHH (British Association for Sexual Health and HIV) (2001) National Guideline on the Management of Vulvovaginal Candidiasis. http://www.bashh.org/guidelines/2002/candida

BASHH (British Association for Sexual Health and HIV) (2002) National Guideline for the Management of Bacterial Vaginosis. http://www.bashh.org/guidelines/2002/bv

BASHH (British Association for Sexual Health and HIV) (2005) United Kingdom National Guideline for the Management of Pelvic Inflammatory Disease (author: Jonathan Ross) http://www.bashh.org/guidelines/2005/pid_v4_0205.doc

Berger BJ, Kolton S, Zenilman JM, Cummins MC, Feldman J, McCormack WM (1995) Bacterial vaginosis in Lesbians: a sexually transmitted disease. *Clinical Infectious Diseases* 21(6) 1402–5

Bevan CD, Johal BJ, Mumtaz G, Ridgway GL, Siddle NC (1995) Clinical, laparoscopic and microbiological findings in acute salpingitis: report on a United Kingdom cohort. *British Journal of Obstricians and Gynaecologists* 102 407–14

DH (Department of Health) (1993) *The Health of the Nation.* DH, London

DH (Department of Health) (2001) *Better Prevention, Better Services, Better Sexual Health – The National Strategy for Sexual Health and HIV.* DH, London

Edwards I, Mason M, Phillips M, Nortonk J, Boyle M (1997) Childhood sexual abuse. Incidence in patients with vulvodynia. *Journal of Reproductive Health* 42/3 135–9

Faculty of Family Planning (2004) The copper Intrauterine Device as a long-term method of contraception. *Journal of Family Planning and Reproductive Health Care* 30/1 29–42

Friedrich EC Jr. (1987) Vulvar vestibulitis syndrome. *Journal of Reproductive Medicine* 38 9–13

Green J, Christmas P, Goldmeir D et al. (2001) A review of physical and psychological factors in vulvar vestibulitis syndrome. *International Journal STD and Aids* 12 705–9

Green Top Guidelines (2000) Investigation and management of endometriosis. www.rog.org.uk/clingov1

Hay PE, Lamont RF, Taylor-Robinson D, Morgan DJ, Ison C, Pearson J (1994) Abnormal bacterial colonisation of the genital tract and subsequent preterm delivery and late miscarriage. *British Medical Journal* 308 295–8

Hillis SD, Joesoef R, Marchbanks PA, Wasserheit JN, Cates W Jr., Westrom L (1993) Delayed care of pelvic inflammatory disease as a risk factor for impaired fertility. *American Journal of Obstetrics and Gynaecology* 168 1503–9

Hurskainen R, Teperi J, Paavonen J, Cacciatore B (1999) Menorrhagia and uterine artery blood flow. *Human Reproduction* 14/1 186–9

International Association for the Study of Pain (1986) in RCOG (2005) *Guideline no 41: Initial Management of Chronic Pain.* RCOG, London

Julius F, Metts MD (1999) Vulvodynia and Vulvar Vestibulitis: Challenges in Diagnosis and Management. *American Family Physician* 59/6 (www.aafp.org)

Kaufman RH, Faro S (1994) in Lotery H, McClure N, Galash R (2004) Vulvodynia. *The Lancet* 363/9414 1058–61

Kinghorn G, Priestly C (1998) Sexually Transmitted Diseases in Shaw R, Soutter W, Stanton S (eds) (1998) *Gynaecology*, 2nd edn. Churchill Livingstone, Edinburgh

Lewis T, Chamberlain G (1999) *Gynaecology by Ten Teachers*. Edward Arnold, London

Lotery H, McClure N, Galash R (2004) Vulvodynia. *The Lancet* 363/9414 1058–61

Lumsden M, Norman J (1998) Menstruation and menstrual abnormality in Shaw R, Soutter W, Stanton S (eds) (1998) *Gynaecology*, 2nd edn. Churchill Livingstone, Edinburgh

McDonald HM, O'Loughlin JA, Vigneswaran R *et al.* (1997) Impact of Metronidazole therapy on preterm birth in women with Bacterial Vaginosis flora: A randomised placebo controlled trial. *British Journal of Obstetrics and Gynaecology* 104 1391–7

Miettinen AK, Heinonen PK, Laippala P, Paavonen J (1993) Test performance of erythrocyte sedimentation rate and C-reactive protein in assessing the severity of acute pelvic inflammatory disease. *American Journal of Obstetrics and Gynecology* 169 1143–9

Mitchell H (2004) Vaginal discharge – Causes, diagnosis and treatment. *British Medical Journal* 328 1306–8

Moore J, Kennedy S, Prentice A (1999) in Green Top Guidelines (2000) Investigation and management of endometriosis, www.rog.org.uk/clingov1

Morcos R, Frost N, Hnat M, Petrunak A, Caldito G (1993) Laparoscopic versus clinical diagnosis of acute pelvic inflammatory disease. *Journal of Reproductive Medicine* 38 53–6

NHS Cervical Screening Programme (1998) *Resource Pack for Training Smear Trainers*. NHS Sheffield

NHS Cervical Screening Programme (2004) *Publication No 20: Colposcopy and Programme Management Guidelines for the NHS Cervical Screening Programmes*. NHS, Sheffield

NHS Cervical Screening Programme (2005) http://www.dh.gov.uk/Home/fs/en

Nugent RP, Krohn MA, Hillier SL (1991) Reliability of diagnosing bacterial vaginosis is improved by a standardized method of Gram stain interpretation. *Journal of Clinical Microbiology* 29 297–301

RCOG (The Royal College of Obstetricians and Gynaecologists) (1998) National Evidence-Based Clinical Guidelines: The Initial Management of Menorrhagia, at www.rcog.org.uk

RCOG (The Royal College of Obstetricians and Gynaecologists) (1999) National Evidence-Based Clinical Guidelines: The Management of Menorrhagia in Secondary Care, at www.rcog.org.uk

RCOG (The Royal College of Obstetricians and Gynaecologists) (2003) *Management of Acute Pelvic Inflammatory Disease* (Guideline No. 32). RCOG, London

RCOG (The Royal College of Obstetricians and Gynaecologists) (2005) *Guideline No. 41: Initial Management of Chronic Pain*. RCOG, London

Sasieni P, Adams J, Cuzick J (2003) Benefits of cervical screening at different ages: evidence from the UK audit of screening histories. *British Journal of Cancer* 89 (July) 88–93 in NHSCSP 2004

Selfe SA, Matthew Z, Stones RW (1998) Benign tumours of the ovary in Shaw R, Soutter W, Stanton S (eds) (1998) *Gynaecology*, 2nd edn. Churchill Livingstone, Edinburgh

Shaw R, Soutter W, Stanton S (eds) (1998) *Gynaecology*, 2nd edn. Churchill Livingstone, Edinburgh

Shaw RW, Soutter WP, Stanton SI (eds) (2003) *Gynaecology*, 3rd edn. Churchill Livingstone, Edinburgh

Silverton L (1993) *The Art and Science of Midwifery*. Prentice-Hall, New York

Simms I, Vickers MR, Stephenson J, Rogers PA, Nicall A (2000) National assessment of PID diagnosis, treatment and management in general practice: England and Wales. *International Journal of STIs and AIDS* 11 440–4

Soutter WP (1998) Benign disease of the vulva and vagina in Shaw R, Soutter W, Stanton S (eds) (1998) *Gynaecology*, 2nd edn. Churchill Livingstone, Edinburgh

Soutter WP, Girling J, Haidopoulos D (2003) Benign tumours of the ovary in Shaw RW, Soutter WP, Stanton SI (2003) *Gynaecology*, 3rd edn, Churchill Livingstone, Edinburgh

Thomas E, Rock J (1997) Endometriosis in Thomas E, Rock J (eds) (1997) *Benign Gynaecological Disease*. Sterling Press, Wellingborough

Turner MI, Marinoff SC (1991) cited in Julius F, Metts MD (1999) Vulvodynia and Vulvar Vestibulitis: Challenges in Diagnosis and Management. *American Family Physician* 59/6 (www.aafp.org)

University of Iowa (1999)

West CP (1998) Uterine Fibroids in Shaw R, Soutter W, Stanton S (eds) (1998) *Gynaecology*, 2nd edn. Churchill Livingstone, Edinburgh

Wisdome A, Hawkins D (1997) *Sexually Transmitted Diseases*, 2nd edn. Mosby Wolfe, London

Yudin MH, Hillier SL, Wiesenfeld HC, Krohn MA, Amortegui AA, Sweet RL (2003) Vaginal polymorphonuclear leucocytes and bacterial vaginosis as markers for histologic endometritis among women without symptoms of pelvic inflammatory disease. *American Journal of Obstetrics and Gynecology* 188/2 318–23

11 Drugs and Pharmacology

SONALI SONECHA

TREATMENT OF GENITO-URINARY PROBLEMS

The choice of treatment is based on a number of factors: effectiveness of therapy, and the cost and availability of the medication. In the United Kingdom, The British Association for Sexual Health and HIV (BASHH) have developed comprehensive guidelines for the treatment and suppression of many common GU problems that are evidence-based. The Centre for Diseases Control (CDC) in the USA also has comprehensive guidelines, with a particularly useful section on the treatment of GUM infections in pregnancy and lactation. This chapter will not look at treatment guidelines, but will focus on the pharmacology of the drugs that are most commonly prescribed in the GUM setting.

INTRODUCTION

Pharmacology is the study of the manner in which the function of living systems is affected by chemical agents (Rang *et al.*, 1999), i.e. it is concerned with the uses, effects and actions of drugs. For a drug to produce a pharmacological response, it would need to 'bind' to the active site (for example, particular constituents of cells or tissues). Most drugs will be bound to protein molecules, although some drugs exert their action by binding to DNA. Once bound, the drug would affect physiological function in a specific manner.

There are four main regulatory proteins that are drug targets:

Receptors: Receptors form the sensing elements in the system of chemical communications that co-ordinates the function of all the different cells in the body (with chemical messengers such as hormones or cytokines, for example). When a drug binds to a receptor it initiates a change in cell function and can cause an effect. If the action of the receptor is activated in this way, then the drug is known as an *agonist*. If the receptor action is inhibited, or the binding of the drug produces no action, then it is known as an *antagonist*.

Enzymes: Enzymes play a major role in the action of drugs. Some drugs are analogues of enzyme substrates. They act by competitively inhibiting the

Advanced Clinical Skills for GU Nurses. Edited by Matthew Grundy-Bowers and Jonathan Davies
© 2007 John Wiley & Sons Ltd

enzyme, and this action can be reversible or irreversible. For example, zidovudine is a thymidine analogue and competitively inhibits the reverse transcriptase enzyme. Other drugs may bind to the enzyme and stop or inhibit its normal function, thereby causing an effect. Some drugs, like valaciclovir, need to undergo metabolism by an enzyme to become active: these are called *pro-drugs*. Sometimes drug toxicity can result, when an enzyme converts a drug molecule into a harmful metabolite.

Carrier molecules: These are responsible for the transport of ions and small organic molecules, such as glucose or amino acids, across cell membranes. The carrier proteins embody a recognition site that makes them specific for a particular permeating species, and these recognition sites can also be targets for drugs whose effect is to block the transport system.

Ion channels: Ion channels are proteins that are found within cell membranes. They control the influx and efflux of ions from the cell. Drugs can act directly or indirectly on ion channels. The simplest mechanism of action is by blocking the ion channel itself, although some drugs may bind to a part of the ion channel and thus modulate its effect. In this way the effect of the ion channel can be either facilitated or impaired.

Drug specificity: For a drug to be useful, it must show specificity for its target-binding site. Specificity is reciprocal: individual classes of drugs bind only to certain targets; individual targets recognise only certain classes of drugs. However, no drug acts with complete specificity. Generally, the lower the potency of a drug, the higher the doses needed to produce an effect, and the more likely it is to bind to active sites other than the one targeted. This may give rise to unwanted side-effects.

GENERAL PRINCIPLES OF PHARMACOKINETICS

Pharmacokinetics is the study of what the body does to the drug. It examines the relationship between drug administration, the time-course of its absorption and distribution throughout the body, and its metabolism and elimination. This is different from pharmacodynamics, which is the study of what the drug does to the body.

ABSORPTION

This is defined as the passage of the drug from its administration site into the plasma. The main routes of administration are:

Oral: The majority of drugs are administered orally, where the drug is absorbed from the gastrointestinal system. Generally, not all of the drug will be absorbed: on average only 75 per cent of an administered dose is absorbed within 3 hours. For some drugs, absorption can be as little as 20 per cent (aciclovir) or as high as almost 100 per cent (doxycycline). There are four main factors that affect gastrointestinal (GI) absorption. These are GI motility and blood flow, GI pH, particle size, and the formulation of the drug and various physiochemical factors (e.g. drug interactions). The fraction of the drug that is absorbed into the systemic circulation and is available at its site of action is known as the bioavailability.

Rectal: This method is useful for drugs that require either local (e.g. glycerine) or systemic (e.g. metronidazole) action. It is a useful alternative in patients who cannot take oral medication and do not have intravenous access. However, absorption can be unreliable.

Injection: Intravenous injection is the fastest method of administration, and results in 100 per cent absorption. Subcutaneous or intramuscular injection of drugs tends to result in faster and greater absorption compared to oral medications. However, the rate of absorption is dependent on the site of the injection, the injection's formulation and the local blood flow.

Application to other epithelial surfaces (e.g. skin, vagina, eye): Topical administration is used whenever a local effect on the skin is required. Generally, most drugs are not absorbed systemically, although this can occasionally happen. For a drug to be absorbed through the skin it would need to be relatively lipid-soluble. Transdermal patches of some drugs are now available, for when a systemic effect is required, for example as a combined contraceptive or for testosterone. Other drug-delivery methods, for example eye drops or vaginal pessaries, are designed for local action, although occasionally systemic absorption can occur.

The sublingual and the inhalatory are the two other main routes of administration employed; however, these are rarely used in GUM.

DISTRIBUTION

The better to understand distribution, it is easier to consider the body as consisting of five main compartments: the plasma, interstitial fluid, intracellular and lymph fluid, transcellular fluid and body fat. Generally, women have less water and more fat then men. How drugs distribute between these compartments is dependent on how lipid-soluble the drug is. The more lipid-soluble the compound the more it will distribute in all compartments and may accumulate in fat. The *blood–brain barrier* is a particularly important entity, and consists of a continuous layer of endothelial cells, joined by tight junctions that ensure that the brain is inaccessible to most compounds, and particularly to poorly lipid-soluble drugs.

Once absorbed, most drugs are distributed in the plasma, either bound to proteins or in 'free' form. Drug molecules that are free are able to move out of the plasma across a cellular barrier towards their target sites. The *volume of distribution (Vd)* is a theoretical measure used to demonstrate how a drug is distributed. It is defined as the volume of plasma that would contain the total body content of the drug at a concentration equal to that in the plasma. The larger the Vd, the more likely the drug is to accumulate outside the plasma.

Understanding how a drug is distributed can allow one to be able to understand better how well a drug will reach its target site. Distribution can vary greatly between individuals and in certain cases: for example, the volume of distribution is increased in pregnancy.

ELIMINATION

Elimination is the irreversible loss of drug from the body. It can occur by two processes. Either the drug is excreted chemically unchanged, or it is metabolised from one chemical entity into another and then removed. The main routes of elimination are the kidneys, the hepatobiliary system (some drugs are excreted in the bile or in faeces) and the lungs.

METABOLISM

Drug metabolism occurs primarily in the liver, by the cytochrome P450 (CYP450) enzyme system. When a drug is absorbed through the GI tract, it often undergoes first-pass metabolism. This is where the absorbed drug passes through the liver before being distributed throughout the rest of the body; and whilst in the liver, it is metabolised. This process can either activate a drug, as is the case with valaciclovir, or form an inactive metabolite, as with the opioid analgesics. Some metabolites may be toxic and lead to adverse effects. If a drug is heavily metabolised in the liver, it can lead to poor oral bioavailablity, resulting in higher doses being required. Some drugs can inhibit or induce CYP450 enzymes, leading to drug–drug interactions. For example, ritonavir is a potent inhibitor of cytochrome isoenzyme 3A4; thus it can greatly affect the bioavailability of other drugs, such as sildenafil.

EXCRETION

The majority of drugs are excreted by the kidneys either unchanged or as metabolites; however, protein-bound drugs will not be renally excreted. In patients with impaired renal function, drug toxicity can sometimes develop if doses are not adjusted. In some cases, the *creatinine clearance (CrCl)* can be calculated for an individual, and can be used to work out the dosing of their drug treatment. Clearance is defined as the volume of plasma containing an amount of substance that is eliminated from the body in a unit of time (ml/min). Generally, the smaller the size of the drug molecule, the more likely it is to be excreted by the kidneys. The liver eliminates some drugs altogether.

However, it is usually much more difficult to gauge liver function, and hence the dosing of drugs is not as straightforward as it otherwise might be.

PREGNANCY AND LACTATION (DONDERS, 2002)

PREGNANCY

There are many issues to consider during pregnancy and breastfeeding.

What is the risk: benefit ratio to the mother and the fetus of treating versus not treating the infection? In some cases – for example, if the woman has a trichomoniasis infection during pregnancy – the morbidity can severely impact on the pregnancy's outcome, so that it would be imperative to treat the infection.

Which trimester of pregnancy is it? Drugs can have a different effect and/or impact on the fetus depending on the stage of pregnancy. For example, non-steroidal agents such as ibuprofen may be harmful to the fetus when given in the final few weeks of pregnancy, as they can cause fetal ductus arteriosus *in utero*.

How long has the drug been on the market? Generally, the longer a product has been licensed, the more data there are available on its safety profile. Many drugs will not be licensed for use in women who are pregnant or breastfeeding, as companies cannot ethically study this, so that most prescribing is based on clinical experience and data from accidental exposure. However, it is a requirement for licensing that potential teratogenicity is studied in animal models, although this does not always correlate with toxicity in humans.

What is the excretion profile of the drug? Not all drugs are excreted in breast milk. For some drugs it may be possible to predict how long after dosing before a drug appears in the breast milk. In this case, the mother may be able to express milk for the infant during the 'safe window'.

What is the age or health of the infant? The same drug may affect the infant differently depending on their age. Infants that are born prematurely may be more sensitive to a drug's effects.

What is the proportion of feeding that is breastfeeding? It is best practice to use drugs that are licensed in pregnancy or lactation where possible, and to always inform the mother of the issues concerned.

USE OF UNLICENSED MEDICINES

Where possible, it is best practice always to use medications that are licensed in the United Kingdom. However, this is not always possible. For example, procaine benzylpenicillin is an antibiotic used as first-line treatment for syphilis in the UK, but is unlicensed and thus needs to be imported from abroad. The

Medicines and Healthcare products Regulatory Agency (MHRA) are responsible for regulating medical products for human use, and they have produced guidance on the usage of unlicensed medications. There are a number of points to consider.

Unlicensed medications need to be ordered on an individual 'named patient' basis. Drugs can be 'named patient' for a number of reasons, for example discontinuation of previously licensed medications or temporary supply problems with UK-licensed versions of a drug, or drugs that are not yet licensed within the UK. The patient should be informed that the medication is unlicensed, without causing undue alarm. It is a legal requirement to maintain records with patient details, prescribing physician, supplier and manufacturer of the product and batch and expiry date of the product. These records need to be held for at least two years.

Any adverse reactions to named-patient drugs can still be reported to the Committee on the Safety of Medicines (CSM) using the yellow-card reporting scheme.

ALLERGIC REACTIONS

Drugs or their reactive metabolites can cause an allergic reaction in patients that may be due to either cell-mediated or antibody-mediated reactions. There are various clinical manifestations of hypersensitivity reactions:

- anaphylaxis, which can be life-threatening when respiration is impaired—most deaths from this are due to penicillin
- haematological reactions – agranulocytosis, haemolytic anaemia or thrombocytopenia – may develop and can sometimes be irreversible
- some patients may have a glucose-6-phosphate dehydrogenase (G6PD) deficiency that can lead to a potentially fatal reaction to some drugs such as sulphonamides
- skin rashes, ranging from very mild to life-threatening (such as Stevens–Johnson syndrome).

Allergy status must always be confirmed and recorded before the administration of any drug, and patients should be informed of any potential signs or symptoms to watch out for if they are at risk of an allergic reaction.

TREATMENT OF ADOLESCENTS

When treating adolescents there are some important considerations: the patient's age and weight can affect the dose of the drug; for example, the dose of hepatitis B vaccine is different for under-15s from the dose for adults. Some drugs may have particular side-effects, making them unsuitable for teenagers: for example, doxycycliney's effects on teeth and bone development. The dosing and administration of treatment should be carefully considered so that minimal disruption is caused to the patient's schooling – for example, dosing three or four times daily or attending the GUM clinic for daily injections may not be feasible. It is important to elicit a full drug history from patients, particularly with regard to alcohol and illicit drug use. The need for parental consent and the patient's need for confidentiality combine to form a complex issue that is covered in another part of this book.

PRACTICAL POINTS ABOUT TAKING AND ADMINISTERING MEDICATIONS

- Some patients may not be able to take certain formulations. Capsules can contain gelatine made from either beef or pork, so that some Jewish, Muslim or Hindu patients will not take these. Other patients may have swallowing difficulties, and require an alternative formulation of the drug.
- Consider the patient's co-morbidities. A number of drugs require dose adjustment in renal or liver impairment. Some gastrointestinal problems may adversely affect the absorption of any GUM treatments prescribed.
- When giving intramuscular injections it is important to ensure that a patient's platelet count is sufficient.
- When taking a drug history from a patient, always check the following:
  - What drugs they are currently taking – including any creams, inhalers, over-the-counter remedies, herbal medicines, recreational drugs and alcohol consumption.
  - In women – pregnancy, lactation and whether they are on hormonal contraception, as the efficacy of it can be affected by some antibiotics.
  - Whether they have recently been on any medication. Some drugs, such as efavirenz (used to treat HIV) are present in significant concentrations in the body for a few weeks after stopping. Other drugs, such as isotretinoin (used to treat severe acne) can still have teratogenic effects up to 3 months after stopping.
  - It is important to check allergy status beforehand. Some patients may not be allergic to the drug itself but to the excipients. For example, naseptin® contains arachis oil, which is not suitable for people with peanut allergy.
  - Some drugs used within GUM have to be used with caution in patients with G6PD deficiency.

ANTIBIOTICS

Antibiotics play a fundamental role in the treatment of sexually transmitted infections. Many centres have their own guidelines, based on resistance patterns seen within the local population, and these guidelines are constantly evolving. There have recently been reports of resistance developing in some populations: for example, to the use of ciprofloxacin in gonorrhoea treatment. GRASP data are collected at a national level to monitor all microbiology samples for trends in the development of drug resistance, seeking to ensure that suboptimal therapy is not being prescribed for gonorrhoea. It is important that, where possible, the choice of treatment for infections is based on individual sensitivities, with consideration also given to local resistance patterns.

Within the genito-urinary medical (GUM) setting, many antibiotics are prescribed as single-dose therapy. The main advantages of this are (a) that it is convenient for the patient and that (b) they can be observed taking their therapy, so that the practitioner can be sure that they have been treated. However, giving higher, single doses may cause more adverse effects and can also potentially have a reduced efficacy in some situations.

Antibiotics can be either bacteriostatic (when the replication of bacterial cells is prevented) or bactericidal (when bacterial cells are killed).

PENICILLINS (RANG *ET AL.*, 1999)

Penicillins belong to the beta-lactam family of antibiotics.

Mode of action

Penicillins work by targeting and binding to the enzymes responsible for bacterial cell-wall synthesis. All pathogenic bacteria possess these enzymes, although the susceptibility of the enzymes can differ, depending on the affinity of the target enzymes to the antibiotic. The action of penicillins can lead to a weakening in the bacterial cell wall, causing lysis (death) of the bacterial cell. However, in some cases this effect can be slow, and thus the penicillin may have a more bacteriostatic effect.

Some bacterial enzymes have acquired resistance to penicillins owing to the production of an enzyme called beta-lactamase that can inactivate penicillins.

Antibacterial activity

Most penicillins have a broad spectrum of activity and can be used against both Gram-negative and Gram-positive organisms. Benzylpenicillin and its long-acting formulations (procaine benzylpenicillin and benzathine penicillin) are particularly active against syphilis. Flucloxacillin is active against *Staphylococcus aureus*, and is often used first-line to treat skin infections. Amoxicillin has a wide range of activity, including action against *Haemophilus influenzae* and *Neisseria gonorrhoee*. The newer generations of penicillins on the market have been designed either to work against β-lactamase-resistant organisms or to have antipseudomonal activity.

Pharmacokinetics

Different penicillins vary in their pharmacokinetics. Amoxicillin has a high oral bioavailability, whereas benzylpenicillin (penicillin G) is so poorly absorbed from the GI tract that it is not available as an oral preparation. Most penicillins can be given by either intravenous or intramuscular injection. Penicillins distribute well in the body; however, they will not cross the blood–brain barrier unless the meninges are inflamed. Penicillins are renally excreted and so will require dose modification in patients with impaired renal function.

Adverse reactions

The majority of patients tolerate penicillins well, the most common adverse effects being mild and gastrointestinal in nature. However, penicillins are also well documented as causing hypersensitivity reactions in some patients, some of which prove to be fatal. If a patient is allergic to one penicillin, then they will also be allergic to the entire class. Additionally, 10 per cent of penicillin-allergic patients will also exhibit an allergy to cephalosporin antibiotics. A skin rash is the most common presenting sign of allergy.

Interactions

Most penicillins do not interact with many other medicines. Probenecid can reduce the renal excretion of some penicillins (by preventing renal tubular secretion), and this interaction is exploited to give higher antibiotic concentrations in the treatment of syphilis (with procaine benzylpenicillin) and gonorrhoea (with amoxicillin).

Treatment of syphilis

Long-acting penicillins (procaine benzylpenicillin G and benzathine penicillin) are the first choice of treatment for most types of syphilis in the UK. They are no longer licensed in the UK, but are available on a 'named patient' basis. High-dose benzylpenicillin is the treatment of choice in patients with tertiary syphilis, or neurosyphilis. Procaine benzylpenicillin is administered by intramuscular injection, and this can be a painful experience for the patient.

Procaine reaction

- This occurs when procaine benzylpenicillin is accidentally administered intravenously.
- Symptoms involve agitation, restlessness, disorientation, tachycardia, nausea, tremors, lethargy and hypotension.
- The toxic reaction is dose-related.

- The patient should be reassured that symptoms will resolve within 30–60 minutes of the administration of the drug.
- If there are any concerns about the patient, medical referral should be made.

Jarisch–Herxheimer reaction

- This is thought to be due to the release of endotoxins from ruptured spirochaetes in patients being treated for syphilis.
- The reaction can affect 50–80 per cent of patients.
- It starts 3–6 hours after administration of the **initial dose** of procaine benzylpenicillin. The reaction will usually resolve within 24 hours.
- Symptoms are flu-like and involve fevers, chills, sore throat, headache, malaise, exacerbation of lesions or outbreak of new lesions. Nausea, vomiting and arthralgia have also been reported.
- Patients should be counselled to take paracetamol for relief of symptoms and be reassured that the reaction is transient.

CEPHALOSPORINS

Cephalosporins are related to penicillins and also belong to the beta-lactam group of antibiotics. There is a 10 per cent cross-sensitivity in allergic patients. Over a hundred different types of cephalosporins are in existence. They are broadly similar, but can differ in bioavailabililty, pharmacokinetics and antibacterial activity.

Antibacterial activity

Cephalosporins are bactericidal, and most cephalosporins have activity against *Staphylococcus aureus*, and Gram-negative *Staphylococci* and *Streptococci*. In the GUM setting, cephalosporins are most commonly used to treat gonorrhoea or urinary tract infections.

Pharmacokinetics

The oral formulations generally have good bioavailability (over 85 per cent), but have relatively short half-lives, and thus require twice- to thrice-daily dosing. They are well distributed, and can achieve high concentrations in the tissues. Most are excreted renally, and so reduced dosing may be necessary in renally impaired patients.

Adverse reactions

For parenteral formulations, pain at the site of injection can be severe, so lidocaine can be added to prevent this, depending on the cephalosporin used. Hypersensitivity can occur in 0.5–10.0 per cent of patients. Gastrointestinal problems are the most common adverse effects, but tend to be mild in nature.

TETRACYCLINES (RANG *ET AL.*, 1999; ZHANEL *ET AL.*, 2004; EMC, 2004A)

Tetracyclines have been around since the 1940s, and are called such because their chemical structure consists of four linear, tetracyclic rings with functional groups attached that differ from one individual agent to the next (Zhanel *et al.*, 2004). They are used in the treatment of many sexually transmitted infections (*Chlamydia*, for example) but their use in treating general bacterial infections has declined in recent years as a result of widespread use in both humans and animals having led to emerging resistance. There are also newer classes of antibiotics now available that have fewer adverse effects and are better tolerated.

Mode of action

Tetracyclines are bacteriostatic antibiotics (although some of the newer atypical tetracyclines are considered to be bactericidal) and work by binding to bacterial ribosomes and inhibiting protein synthesis within the bacterial cell.

Antibacterial activity

Tetracyclines have a broad spectrum of activity and are useful against both Gram-positive and Gram-negative bacteria as well as some atypical organisms such as *Mycoplasma*, *Chlamydia*, spirochetes and some protozoa. Doxycycline (vibramycin) can even be used in malaria prevention. In GU medicine, doxycycline is the most commonly used tetracycline, for example in the treatment of syphilis or *Chlamydia*.

Pharmacokinetics

Tetracyclines are available in both oral and parenteral forms. Different tetracyclines have varying degrees of bioavailability when taken orally, and doxycycline is virtually completely absorbed from the gastrointestinal tract and is unaffected by food or milk intake. It distributes throughout the body and can cross the placenta in pregnant women. Tetracyclines can be excreted either in the bile or by the kidneys (they may thus require dose adjustments in renal impairment). Doxycycline is highly protein-bound, and the bulk of its excretion is in the bile.

Adverse effects

The most common adverse effects are gastrointestinal in nature. It is recommended that doxycycline be taken with water whilst standing or sitting to minimise oesophageal ulceration. Tetracyclines are deposited in growing bones and teeth, sometimes causing staining or affecting development. For this reason they are not recommended in pregnancy or lactation or in growing children. Phototoxicity (causing sunburn-type symptoms) has been reported in patients on tetracyclines. Patients should be advised to stay out of the sun or to use sunblock whilst on the drug, and to avoid sunbeds too. Rare adverse effects include blood dyscrasias, hepatotoxicity and discoloration of teeth under long-term treatment.

Interactions

Tetracyclines chelate with metal ions such as calcium or iron, and for this reason should not be administered with antacids or iron preparations, as these will reduce absorption. Patients can be advised to dose at least two hours apart if taking both. Tetracyclines, being bacteriostatic, may also interfere with the bactericidal effects of penicillins, so that care should be taken when using the two together.

FLUOROQUINOLONE ANTIBIOTICS (RANG *ET AL.*, 1999; EMC, 2003)

Quinolone antibiotics include ciprofloxacin and ofloxacin and are used in GU medicine to treat a variety of infections.

Mode of action

Quinolones are bactericidal and act by inhibiting bacterial DNA gyrase enzymes, thereby interfering with bacterial DNA function.

Antibacterial activity

Ciprofloxacin and ofloxacin are broad-spectrum antibiotics with activity against Gram-positive and especially Gram-negative organisms. They are also active against some anaerobes and *Chlamydia* and *Mycoplasma* species. Since their launch, quinolones have been widely used, and this has led to the emergence of resistance in some bacterial species. This has been seen in the GUM setting, where in some geographical areas in the UK the increasing amount of gonorrhoea resistant to ciprofloxacin has led to its no longer being considered as a first-line empirical treatment in local guidelines for this condition.

Pharmacokinetics

Quinolones are well absorbed when taken orally; ciprofloxacin has a bioavailability of 70–80 per cent. Ciprofloxacin is affected by the cytochrome P450 enzyme system in the liver, and thus has a number of important drug interactions. Most quinolones either undergo hepatic metabolism or renal excretion or a mixture of the two.

Adverse effects

Ciprofloxacin is generally well tolerated, and most side-effects tend to be gastrointestinal and mild in nature. In some patients, ciprofloxacin can cause central nervous system effects that can affect patients' ability to carry out tasks that require concentration, such as driving.

Interactions

Absorption of ciprofloxacin can be reduced if it is taken at the same time as dairy products, antacid or iron preparations; ciprofloxacin should be dosed at least four hours apart from these products. Quinolones can inhibit the cytochrome P450 system, and thus interact with a number of different drugs. Some of these interactions can be potentially serious: for example, ciprofloxacin can cause an increase in theophylline levels, potentially leading to toxicity.

MACROLIDE ANTIBIOTICS (RANG *ET AL.*, 1999)

Erythromycin was the first macrolide to be developed, and has been a mainstay of treatment for many infections for the last forty years. More recently clarithromycin and azithromycin have become available in the UK. Their main benefits are that they offer easier dosing, are more tolerable to take and do not have as many drug interactions.

Mechanism of action

Macrolides can be either bactericidal or bacteriostatic, depending on the concentration of the drug and the type of micro-organism involved. They work by binding to the bacterial ribosome, and thus preventing protein synthesis.

Antibacterial activity

All three macrolides are broad-spectrum and cover similar organisms to penicillin, and for this reason are often used to treat infections in penicillin-allergic patients. They are more effective against Gram-positive organisms than Gram-negative ones. Additionally, clarithromycin and azithromycin can be used to treat *Mycoplasma* infections such as the *Mycobacterium avium* complex (an opportunistic infection in AIDS patients).

Pharmacokinetics

All three macrolides have good oral bioavailability and diffuse into most tissues. However, they do not have as good CSF penetration as the beta-lactam antibiotics. Erythromycin has a short plasma half-life of around 90 minutes; hence it is generally dosed four times daily. Clarithromycin and azithromycin both have much longer half-lives. Azithromycin is converted in the liver to an active metabolite, and persists in tissues at high concentrations; thus it has the advantage of being able to be given as a single dose for some infections, allowing for directly observed therapy and assurance that the patient has taken the appropriate treatment. Azithromycin capsules need to be taken on an empty stomach, and should be dosed separately from iron or indigestion remedies. Azithromycin tablets are also available; these are 500 mg (as opposed to 250 mg) capsules, and do not have any food restrictions. All three macrolides are excreted in the bile.

Adverse effects

Most side-effects are gastrointestinal. Erythromycin in particular can cause nausea and vomiting in some patients. Clarithromycin and azithromycin are tolerated better, and are good alternatives in patients who are intolerant of erythromycin. Some patients are allergic to macrolides, and a hypersensitivity to one macrolide confers cross-class allergy. Erythromycin has also been known to cause reversible hearing loss. Erythromycin is safe to use in pregnancy and lactation. Azithromycin is not licensed in the UK for use in pregnancy; however, some GUM centres use it in pregnancy following a detailed discussion with the mother-to-be.

Interactions

All macrolides go through first-pass metabolism in the liver, and as such are susceptible to interacting with other drugs that also pass through the cytochrome P450 system. Erythromycin has the most interactions of the three.

METRONIDAZOLE (RANG *ET AL.*, 1999; FINCH *ET AL.*, 2003; KINGSTON & CARLIN, 2002; EMC, 2005A)

Metronidazole belongs to a class of antibiotics called Nitroimidazoles.

Mechanism of action

Metronidazole is bactericidal, and works by binding to the DNA of the micro-organism and causing strand breakage.

Antibacterial activity

Metronidazole is active against anaerobic bacteria, microaerophilic species and some protozoa. In GUM it is most often used in the treatment of bacterial vaginosis, *Trichomonas vaginalis* or *Giardia*.

Pharmacokinetics

Metronidazole is well absorbed from the GI tract and distributes well throughout the body. It has a half-life of approximately 8 hours, and thus requires dosing two to three times daily.

Unwanted effects

The most common effects are GI disturbances such as nausea or diarrhoea. Metronidazole can also leave a metallic taste in the mouth. It is best taken with or after food and with a glass of water to minimise these effects.

Interactions

Metronidazole can interact with alcohol, causing a disulfram-like reaction. Patients should be advised to avoid all alcohol (including any in food) whilst on therapy and for two days after finishing the course.

CLINDAMYCIN (RANG *ET AL.*, 1999; FINCH *ET AL.*, 2003; EMC, 2004B)

Clindamycin belongs to a small, novel class of antibiotics called lincosamides. Clindamycin is a semi-synthetic version of a naturally occurring antibiotic, and the only one in its class that is licensed in the UK for use in humans.

Mechanism of action

Clindamycin inhibits protein synthesis in bacterial cells in a similar fashion to macrolides.

Antibacterial activity

Clindamycin is active against Gram-positive organisms and anaerobes and some mycoplasmas and protozoans, but not against Gram-negative organisms.

It has good activity against *Staphylococcius* and *Streptococcus* organisms. In GUM, clindamycin is most often used to treat bacterial vaginosis (caused by an overgrowth of local anaerobic bacteria in the vaginal flora).

Pharmacokinetics

Clindamycin is well absorbed and distributes well in the body, including soft tissues and bone. It is largely metabolised by the liver and excreted in the bile. When administered vaginally, it has a local effect, with only a minimal amount being absorbed systemically.

Unwanted effects

Clindamycin can cause gastrointestinal upset in some patients and can occasionally cause rashes. Its most well-known adverse effect is having the potential to cause the *Clostridium difficile* diarrhoea that can lead to the potentially fatal pseudomembranous colitis. For this reason it is imperative to counsel patients to discontinue clindamycin immediately if they develop diarrhoea, and to seek medical advice right away.

Interactions

Clindamycin for vaginal use can weaken the rubber of condoms and diaphragms. Patients should be advised to use an alternative method of contraception whilst on treatment.

TRIMETHOPRIM (RANG *ET AL.*, 1999; FINCH *ET AL.*, 2003)

Trimethoprim belongs to a class of antibiotics called diaminopyrimidines (antifolates), and is the most commonly used antibiotic in its class. It has been used in the clinical setting for the last thirty years.

Mechanism of action

Trimethoprim is a potent inhibitor of the enzyme dihydrofolate reductase, i.e. it acts as a folate antagonist. Bacteria use folates as part of the process of DNA or RNA synthesis, and inhibiting this process will inhibit bacterial growth. Thus its action is bacteriostatic.

Antibacterial activity

Trimethoprim is a broad-spectrum agent with activity against Gram-positive bacilli and cocci, enterobacteria and some other non-bacterial organisms. In the UK trimethoprim is mainly used to treat urinary tract infections. However, resistance to trimethoprim is increasing in the UK. Trimethoprim is also combined with sulfamethoxazole (co-trimoxazole), which plays an important role in the prevention and treatment of some HIV-related opportunistic infections.

Pharmacokinetics

Trimethoprim is almost completely absorbed from the GI tract, and has a plasma half-life of 8 to 11 hours, allowing for twice-daily dosing. It is well distributed in the body and into the CSF, kidneys and lungs. It can cross the placenta and is excreted in breast milk. Most of the drug is excreted unchanged in the urine; thus dose reduction is required in patients with impaired renal function.

Adverse effects

The most common side-effects are nausea and vomiting. Rarely, patients may develop skin rashes or are allergic to trimethoprim, and in some cases they may suffer from haematological side-effects.

Interactions

Trimethoprim may interact with warfarin and rifampicin. It should be used cautiously with other drugs that are bone-marrow depressants.

ANTIVIRAL AGENTS (LEUNG & SACKS, 2000)

ACICLOVIR (FINCH *ET AL.*, 2003; RANG *ET AL.*, 1999)

Aciclovir was one of the first specific inhibitors of antiviral activity and is virastatic inaction.

Mechanism of action

Aciclovir is a purine nucleoside analogue of guanosine. It acts by terminating DNA chain synthesis and inhibits DNA polymerase. It is extremely specific in its activity, as it needs to be phosphorylated in the cell before it can be used by the **viral** enzyme thymidine kinase.

Antiviral activity

Aciclovir is active against *Herpes simplex* virus (HSV) types 1 and 2 and against *Varicella zoster* virus. It is not generally active against other viruses. It can be used both for treatment of acute attacks and in suppression.

Pharmacokinetics

Aciclovir is poorly absorbed (~20 per cent of dose) from the GI tract. It has a half-life of only three hours; hence the necessity for frequent dosing when given orally. Aciclovir is widely distributed in the body, including into the CSF and vesicular fluid. It can cross the placenta and is excreted into breast milk. Aciclovir is excreted unchanged in the urine, and so requires dose-reduction in patients with renal impairment.

Unwanted effects

Patients may occasionally exhibit a form of contact dermatitis in response to the cream. Common side-effects of oral aciclovir include headache and nausea. A small minority of patients are allergic to aciclovir. The primary disadvantage of aciclovir is that its frequency of dosing may lead to impaired adherence. This could in turn lead to the development of resistant virus.

Interactions

Aciclovir does not interact with many other drugs.

VALACICLOVIR (LEUNG & SACKS, 2000)

This is a pro-drug of aciclovir, and as such has the same mechanism of action, spectrum of antiviral activity, adverse effects and interactions. Patients who are allergic to aciclovir will also be allergic to valaciclovir.

Pharmacokinetics

Valaciclovir is the L-valyl ester of aciclovir. It has a much higher bioavailability (~60%) than aciclovir. Valaciclovir is easily absorbed from the GI tract and almost completely converted to aciclovir. This means that it can be dosed less frequently than aciclovir. Valaciclovir is excreted via the kidneys in the same way as aciclovir.

FAMCICLOVIR

Famciclovir is also a synthetic purine nucleoside analogue.

Mechanism of action

Famciclovir also inhibits viral DNA synthesis. It too requires phosphorylation before it can be effective against viruses. Famciclovir works by acting as a substrate inhibitor for viral DNA polymerase. It has less affinity for DNA polymerase than aciclovir, but higher intracellular concentrations.

Antiviral activity

Famciclovir has a similar spectrum of activity to aciclovir.

Pharmacokinetics

Famciclovir is a pro-drug that is converted to penciclovir in the body. Penciclovir is virtually unabsorbed orally, whereas famciclovir has a bioavailability of approximately 75 per cent. The intracellular half-life of penciclovir is approximately 20 hours, and so it can be dosed less frequently than aciclovir. Its primary route of excretion is renal.

Unwanted effects

Famciclovir is similar to aciclovir. Patients who are allergic to aciclovir may also exhibit allergy to famciclovir.

ANTIFUNGAL AGENTS

Antifungal agents are used in the GUM setting mainly to treat *Candida* spp.

FLUCONAZOLE

Fluconazole belongs to a group of agents called the azoles.

Mechanism of action

Fluconazole is a triazole antifungal. Triazole refers to the fact that the structure of fluconazole contains three imidazole rings. Azoles work by blocking the synthesis of ergosterol, which is used in the production of fungal cell membranes. The action of fluconazole is fungistatic.

Antifungal activity

Fluconazole is active against dermatophytes, dimorphic fungi and some yeasts (such as *Candida*).

Pharmacokinetics

Fluconazole is almost completely absorbed when given orally. It has a half-life of 25 to 30 hours, so can be dosed once daily. Fluconazole is widely distributed in the body fluids and tissues. It is excreted mostly unchanged in the urine, and thus dose adjustment is required in patients with renal impairment.

Unwanted effects

Fluconazole is generally well tolerated. It can cause GI side-effects such as nausea and diarrhoea. Rarely it can cause liver enzyme abnormalities or serious skin reactions.

CLOTRIMAZOLE

Clotrimazole is also part of the azole class. In GUM it is used as a topical agent to treat a variety of fungal dermatological infections.

Mechanism of action

Clotrimazole has a similar mechanism of action to fluconazole. However, as it is present in higher concentrations, it is fungicidal.

Antifungal activity

Topical clotrimazole can be used to treat a variety of dermatophytes and *Candida*.

Pharmacokinetics

When used as a cream or as a pessary, clotrimazole has a local effect and does not get absorbed into the systemic circulation.

Unwanted effects

Some patients may be hypersensitive to clotrimazole or other imidazoles. Occasionally, patients may get some local irritation from clotrimazole.

Interactions

Clotrimazole when used with latex contraceptives can reduce their efficacy. Patients should be advised to use alternative methods of contraception or to abstain from sexual intercourse whilst on treatment.

TREATMENT OF WARTS

Condylomata acuminata (genital warts) are benign proliferative tumours, and are caused by human papilloma viruses (HPV). These are double-stranded DNA viruses that infect squamous epithelial cells. There are different types of HPV, which can be either low-risk (can cause genital warts) or high-risk (can cause cancers). Most patients that are infected with HPV will remain unsymptomatic; however, a small minority of patients will develop genital warts. Immunocompromised patients are more likely to develop systemic infections due to HPV. Disease symptoms can be physically painful and can cause considerable psychological distress.

PODOPHYLLOTOXIN (EMC, 2005B)

Podophyllotoxin is the purified form of podophyllin, an antimitotic agent, and it is a chemical, topical treatment that is used to remove genital warts.

Mechanism of action

Podophyllotoxin works by binding to tubulin and preventing cell division (mitosis), and thereby inhibiting growth of the viral cells.

Points to note

Patients should be counselled to wash and dry affected areas before applying podophyllotoxin and to take care not to get it on to any unaffected skin.

Some patients may experience local irritation after starting treatment. This tends to be mild, and will sometimes decrease with time. Podophyllotoxin is not absorbed into the systemic circulation.

IMIQUIMOD (PERRY & LAMB, 1999)

Imiquimod belongs to a new class of drugs called immune response modifiers.

Mode of action

Imiquimod is an imidazoquinoline, and its antiviral activity is mediated by its ability to stimulate the production of interferon alpha and other cytokines in HPV-infected cells, thereby mediating an immune response to HPV. Studies have shown that clearance of warts correlates with a lower viral load in wart tissue.

Pharmacokinetics

Pharmacokinetic data on imiquimod are limited. However, it is not thought to be absorbed systemically through the skin or through genital tissue.

Adverse effects

Imiquimod is generally well tolerated and does not tend to show any systemic adverse effects. Over half the patients treated in studies have shown some form of local skin irritation, such as erythema, itching and burning. These tend to be mild, and cause discontinuation in only 1–2 per cent of patients. There has been hypopigmentation or hyperpigmentation reported in some patients, and it is unclear whether this is permanent or reversible. It is important to note that there have been reports of severe reactions at the urethral meatus, causing dysuria in women (EMC, 2004c).

Interactions

As a topical preparation, imiquimod has limited systemic absorption, and it is not known to interact with many medications. However, the cream can weaken diaphragms and condoms (EMC, 2004c), so patients should be advised to use alternative forms of contraception whilst using the cream.

REFERENCES

Donders GGG (2002) Treatment of sexually transmitted bacterial diseases in pregnant women. *Drugs* 59(3) (March) 477–85

Electronic Medicines Compendium (2003) Summary of Product Characteristics for Ciproxin, last updated 13 November

Electronic Medicines Compendium (2004a) Summary of Product Characteristics for Vibramycin, last updated 26 October 2004

Electronic Medicines Compendium (2004b) Summary of Product Characteristics for Clindamycin, last updated 28 September 2004

Electronic Medicines Compendium (2004c) Summary of Product Characteristics for Aldara 5% cream, last updated 4 August

Electronic Medicines Compendium (2005a) Summary of Product Characteristics for Flagyl, last updated 27 September

Electronic Medicines Compendium (2005b) Summary of Product Characteristics for podophyllotoxin, last updated 27 September

Finch RG, Greenwood D, Norrby SR, Whitley RJ (eds) (2003) *Antibiotic and Chemotherapy: Anti-infective Agents and Their Use in Therapy*, 8th edn. Churchill Livingstone, Edinburgh

Kingston M, Carlin E (2002) Treatment of sexually transmitted infections with single dose therapy: a double-edged sword. *Drugs* 62(6) 871–8

Leung DT, Sacks SL (2000) Current Recommendations for the Treatment of Genital Herpes. *Drugs* 60(6) 1329–52

Perry CM, Lamb HA (1999) Topical Imiquimod: A review of its use in genital warts. *Drugs* 58(2) (August) 375–90

Rang HP, Dale MM, RitterJM (eds) (1999) *Pharmacology*, 4th edn. Churchill Livingstone, Edinburgh

Zhanel GG *et al.* (2004) The Glycylcyclines: A comparative review with the tetracyclines. *Drugs* 64(1) 63–88

12 Patient Group Directions and Nurse Prescribing

CINDY GILMOUR AND JANE BICKFORD

INTRODUCTION

The meeting of an individual's healthcare needs is traditionally undertaken by a doctor using a process of assessment, diagnosis and review, which may also include the prescribing of appropriate medication. This is a typical outline of a general management plan, particularly with regard to chronic healthcare needs. Today this concept of care is gradually changing owing to the evolution and development of professional roles – healthcare professionals other than doctors are now able to manage patients independently by utilising their clinical skills and knowledge and expertise in order to make effective interventions and safe decisions about patient care. This can be demonstrated within the realm of sexual health, where in the past ten years nursing roles have developed to meet the ever-changing needs of those attending sexual health clinics, including the development of the roles of Nurse Consultants and Nurse Practitioners/Specialist Nurses. Facilitation of these role progressions into independent practice and autonomy has been aided by the use of patient group directions (formerly known as group protocols) and the ability to undertake independent and supplementary prescribing. The use of patient group directions in particular has greatly enhanced patient care within sexual health and has led to many innovative services, particularly in Outreach settings, for instance hepatitis A and B vaccinations for gay and bisexual men.

This chapter will now present an overview of the development of patient group directions in relation to legislation and application to practice, as well as discussing independent and supplementary prescribing, including the required knowledge and competencies.

EVOLUTION OF PATIENT GROUP DIRECTIONS

Patient group directions were formerly known as 'group protocols', and were derived from recommendations contained within the first Crown Report (DH,

Advanced Clinical Skills for GU Nurses. Edited by Matthew Grundy-Bowers and Jonathan Davies
© 2007 John Wiley & Sons Ltd

1989). Primarily this Crown Report focused upon recommendations and criteria for the authorisation of nurses working in the community (who held District Nurse and/or Health Visiting qualifications) to be able to prescribe medicines from a limited Nurse Prescribers' Formulary (NPF). However, the view was also advocated that doctors and nurses, in collaboration, could produce group protocols using local guidance in the administering and supplying of medicines (McHale, 2003). As more and more emphasis was being applied to 'patient-centred care', group protocols were seen as a potential benefit to the development of hospital services by providing quicker access to treatment, reducing waiting times and, most importantly, efficiently utilising and enhancing existing resources and professional skills (DH, 1998). Examples of where group protocols were initially used included travel and flu vaccination services (NPC, 2004).

Over time, though, concerns became raised around the actual legalities of using group protocols for the supply and administration of medicines, and whether patient safety was being compromised. Some of these concerns included the legal acceptability of nurses administering medication to patients who had not been seen by a medical practitioner, and working under group protocols that related to groups of patients rather than being patient-specific (McHale, 2003). In response, the Department of Health (DH) commissioned a review of supplying and administering medicines under group protocols which was led by June Crown in 1998, and resulted in the publication of the second Crown Report Part 1 (DH, 1998).

The Crown Report defines a group protocol as:

> ... a specific written instruction for the supply or administration of named medicines in an identified clinical situation. It is drawn up locally by doctors, pharmacists and other appropriate professionals, and approved by the employer, advised by the relevant professional advisory committees. It applies to groups of patients or other service users who may not be individually identified before presentation for treatment (Crown Report 1998 Appendix E: DH, 1998).

The Advisory Group found, on reviewing existing group protocols, many anomalies regarding the written interpretation and implementation of group protocols within clinical practice. Inconsistencies were evident with regard to the monitoring, authorisation, responsibility and accountability of group protocols, and importantly there appeared a lack of clarity surrounding the actual requirements needed for the clinical criteria and types of medicines being used (DH, 1998).

In order to aid the process of clarification, the Advisory team produced criteria to support the development of group protocols and gave current and future recommendations for the conformity and standardisation of all current and future group protocols within established and legal criteria. In particular, the Advisory team recommended that 'the majority of patients should continue to receive medicines on an individual basis. However, there is likely to be a continuing need for supply and administration under group protocols in certain limited situations as part of a comprehensive health service and most importantly '*the law should be clarified to ensure that health professionals who supply or administer medicines under approved protocols are acting within the law*' (NHS Executive, 1998: HSC 1998/051, P. 4).

Following this in-depth review and subsequent recommendations outlined in the Crown Report Part 1 (DH, 1998), a consultation document (referred to as MLX 260) was issued in March 2000 by the Medicines and Healthcare Products Regulatory Agency (MHRA), entitled *Sale, supply and administration of medicines by health professionals under patient group directions* (MHRA, 2000). Within this document, the terminology changed, and 'group protocol' was now referred to as '*patient group direction*'. Proposed amendments were outlined with regard to the Medicines Act 1968 and other medicine regulations, which would then in turn allow nurses and other healthcare professionals specifically to use patient group directions (PGDs) within agreed legal criteria. Other proposals for consideration included suggested mechanisms for approving PGDs, the use or exemption of certain controlled and unlicensed medicines within PGDs and identification of areas within the NHS and private sector where PGDs could be implemented (MHRA, 2000).

A definition of a PGD was also given in the document issued by the MHRA that was very similar to the existing definition of a group protocol, and read:

> . . . a specific written instruction for the supply and administration, or administration of a named medicine in an identified clinical situation. This definition applies to presenting for groups of patients who may not be individually identified before presenting for treatment. Patient group directions are drawn up locally by doctors, pharmacists and other health professionals, signed by a doctor or a dentist, as appropriate and approved by an appropriate healthcare body' (MHRA, 2000, p. 2)

It may be prudent here to mention the term 'patient specific direction' – this is where a prescriber (doctor, dentist or nurse) directs another healthcare worker to administer or supply medicines to a named patient(s) (NPC, 2004). It is important to have an understanding of both of these terms in order to allay any confusion and potential misunderstanding surrounding the legal requirements for the administration and supply of medicines.

In considering the proposed amendments to satisfy legal requirements, the consultation document (MLX 260: MHRA, 2000) included a regulatory appraisal that listed four possible options, and outcomes (Table 17) that could potentially impact upon the future use of patient group directions.

Following consultation, Option 3 was the most favoured, as it was deemed appropriate enough to allow current effective practice to continue without compromising patient safety and also it would maximise the efficient use of resources and clinical skills in practice. It was also suggested that this option would not greatly impact upon costing in terms of producing new PGDs to satisfy the new legal requirements.

Table 17

Options put forward by MHRA consultation document mlx 260 (MHRA, 2000)

Option 1 – Do nothing.
Option 2 – Voluntary agreement by appropriate healthcare sectors to ensure
directions meet the standards recommended in the Crown report, supplemented
by centrally issued guidance.
Option 3 – Amend the law as proposed to remove uncertainty about the legality of
the operation of group directions and set out legal criteria that they will need to
meet. This option would interpret the law more widely and allow for directions to
apply to unnamed groups of patients with a particular clinical condition.
Option 4 – Amend the law to confirm existing views on the meaning of 'directions'.
This option would result in a narrower interpretation of the existing law, as group
directions that did not apply to named patients would be illegal.

In context then, from the initial recommendations of the Crown Report Part
1 (DH, 1998) and the response to the MHRA consultation document (MLX
260), a Health Circular was issued in 2000 to all chief executives, which contained amended legislative requirements and guidance pertaining to the use
of PGDs (NHS Executive, 2000: HSC 2000/026). Changes were made accordingly to The Prescription Only Medicines (Human Use) Amendment Order
2000, the Medicine (Pharmacy and General Sale – Exemption) Amendment
Order 2000 and the Medicines (Sale and Supply) (Miscellaneous provisions)
Amendment (No. 2) – these amendments are legally defined within the Statutory Instruments 2000 Nos. 1917, 1919 and 1918 respectively.

To further clarify the appropriate use of PGDs the NHS Executive stated
that:

> *The majority of clinical care should be provided on an individual, patient specific*
> *basis. The supply and administration of medicines under patient group directions*
> *should be reserved for those limited situations where this offers an advantage for*
> *patient care (without compromising patient safety) and where it is consistent with*
> *appropriate professional relationships and accountability* (NHS Executive, 2000:
> 2000/026 p. 2).

DEVELOPING A PATIENT GROUP DIRECTION (PGD)

Information that needs to be specified within the development of a PGD is
clearly defined within HSC 2000/026 (see Table 18), and it is imperative that
this information is integrated into existing PGDs and complied with in order
for the PGD to be lawful.

In order to help the reader gain a clearer perception and understanding in
writing and devising a PGD, the legislative framework encompassed within
the Crown Report (DH, 1998) and HSC 2000/026 (NHS Executive, 2000) will

Table 18 Legislative requirements for the date that must be contained
within each PGD (NHS Executive 2000)

- The name of the business to which the direction applies
- The date the direction comes into force and the date it expires
- A description of the medicine(s) to which the direction applies
- The class of health professional who may supply or administer the medicine
- Signature of a doctor or dentist, as appropriate, and pharmacist
- Signature by the appropriate health organisation
- The clinical condition or situation to which the direction applies
- A description of those patients excluded from treatment under the direction
- A description of the circumstances in which further advice should be sought from a doctor (or dentist as appropriate) and arrangements for referral
- Details of appropriate dosage and maximum total dosage, quantity, pharmaceutical form and strength, route and frequency of administration, and minimum or maximum period over which the medicine should be administered
- Relevant warnings, including potential adverse reactions
- Details of any necessary follow-up action and circumstances
- A statement of the records to be kept for audit purposes

be discussed in more depth. Some areas will be illustrated in tables (Tables 19, 20 and 21) with reference to a current PGD used by the authors for the administration and supply of medication for the treatment of genital candidiasis (Gilmour *et al.*, 2005).

The comprehensive criteria contained within the 1998 Crown Report that underpin the formulation of a PGD are divided into 3 sections:

- Content
- Development
- Implementation.

CONTENT OF A PATIENT GROUP DIRECTION

This section refers to the clinical conditions that apply to the PGD, the characteristics of the staff that are authorised to administer and supply medicines, the description of the treatment available and the management and monitoring of PGDs.

- ***Clinical condition*** – The clinical condition or situation to which the PGD pertains must be clearly stated. Inclusion and exclusion criteria must be established, as well as detailing actions and information necessary to deal with those patients excluded from the PGD, as well as those patients who decline treatment. These actions and any other information given must be clearly documented within the patient notes.
- ***Characteristics of staff authorised to take responsibility for the supply or administration of medicines under Patient Group Direction*** – Up to May

Table 19

Clinical condition, inclusion and exclusion criteria for the treatment of genital candidiasis

Clinical condition – The PGD is applicable to any patient (male or female) who has been diagnosed with genital candidiasis. Genital candidiasis is a fungal infection and is commonly caused by the species *Candida albicans*. In women the sites of infection may include the vulva, vagina and the urethra, and in men the most common sites include the glans, prepuce and urethra. Signs and symptoms are variable. Women may complain of a thick white vaginal discharge, pruritus, soreness, erythema, dysuria and dyspareunia. Fissuring may be apparent on the vulva. Men may present with a visible rash on the glans and they may also complain of pruritus and dysuria. Diagnosis is confirmed either clinically, microscopically (by wet and dry slide) or by culture media.

Inclusion criteria – symptomatic patients who have had *Candida* diagnosed clinically and/or microscopically, and symptomatic patients who have had *Candida* diagnosed on culture.

Exclusion criteria – this includes female patients who have *Candida* diagnosed microscopically or on culture but are asymptomatic, female patients who have recurrent vulvovaginal candidiasis (RVVC*) as denoted by 4 or more mycologically proven symptomatic episodes in the previous 12 months, patients who have any known allergy to any constituents found within the medication, women who are pregnant/breastfeeding and who require fluconazole and patients with co-existing renal or hepatic disease who require fluconazole.

*For patients considered to have RVVC they will be referred to a consultant specialist clinic (as per clinic guidelines), and all other patients excluded from treatment will be referred to a doctor within the clinic. The nurse will offer a referral to a doctor – if this is declined the nurse will document the discussion, and the decision made by the patient to decline treatment.
Source: Gilmour, C. *et al*. 2005.

Table 20

Competencies required to undertake treatment of genital candidiasis

For the supply of medication for genital candidiasis it is not only important that the nurse has a full understanding of the physiological disease process of *Candida* and awareness of differential diagnoses, but is also competent in taking a comprehensive sexual history as well as general medical history, providing clear and current health education, recognising dermatological conditions which can mimic candidiasis and having the ability to diagnose candida clinically and microscopically.

To be able to supply treatment under the PGD – the nurse will be expected to:

- Understand the indications and contra-indications for the use of the medicines specified
- Be aware of the route and method of administration
- Be aware of the potential side-effects and discuss with patient
- Have an understanding of the potential drug interactions

Source: Gilmour, C. *et al*. 2005.

Table 21

Information to be included for audit purposes

An audit tool will be developed ... in order to provide a clear audit trail – the first audit of notes will be done three months after working to the patient group direction for the treatment of genital candidiasis. A sample of notes will be reviewed for documented evidence of:

- Appropriate diagnosis
- Correct inclusion criteria for treatment
- Possible contraindications excluded
- Appropriate treatment given
- Correct documentation of treatment supplied/administered
- Advice given to clients

A sample of notes (at least 20 or 50% of the patients seen) will be audited yearly. A short summary will be written within four weeks of its taking place. This must be clearly signed and dated by the nurse using the PGD and the consultant mentor.

Source: Gilmour, C. *et al*. 2005.

2004 the following qualified professionals were able to use PGDs – nurses, midwives, health visitors, optometrists, pharmacists, chiropodists, radiographers, orthoptists, physiotherapists and ambulance paramedics. Changing legislation from May 2004 now allows other qualified professionals, including dietitians, occupational therapists, prosthetists and orthotists and speech and language therapists to use PGDs.

The required level of specialist knowledge and training and the level of competency expected should be clearly stated within the PGD – not only with regard to the clinical condition, but also to the knowledge of the medicines being used. It is also important to document episodes of supervised practice with a medical mentor and to have a written agreement that the individual using the PGD possesses all the relevant competencies to supply and administer medication effectively without compromising patient care and safety. For reference, a list of individuals deemed competent to use certain PGDs should be held locally within the organisation. The recognised training and qualifications will differ according to local NHS Trust, Health Authority or Primary Care Trust (PCT) policy. It is also important to stress that an individual can only use a PGD to administer and supply medicines as a *named individual* within the PGD.

- *Description of treatment available under the PGD* – this section includes the names and the legal status of all medicines that will be used within the PGD.

From The Medicines Act 1968, medicines are allocated into 3 categories as described by the MHRA (2005):

- Prescription Only Medicines (POM) – these medicines can only be sold or supplied at registered pharmacy premises, and in accordance with an appropriate practitioner's prescription.
- Pharmacy Medicines (P) – medicines that can be sold or supplied at a registered pharmacy under the supervision of a pharmacist.
- General Sales List (GSL) – these medicines can be bought from a number of premises, including supermarkets, as long as the medicines are pre-packed and the premises are lockable to the general public.

Other categories of medicines that need to be considered with regard to use within a PGD include unlicensed and controlled medicines.

Unlicensed medicines are currently excluded from PGDs, but recent legislation has allowed the inclusion of Black Triangle Drugs and medicines used outside the terms of the Summary of Product Characteristics (RCN, 2004). The Summary of Product Characteristics (SPC) relates to the data sheets that accompany each drug. Black triangle drugs are recently licensed drugs and vaccines that are being closely monitored for any adverse reactions, and are usually subject to special reporting procedures (usually for a minimum period of two years). Their use within a PGD must be justified within the remit of best clinical practice, and it must be clearly stated within the PGD that a black triangle drug is being used or that a product is being used outside the SPC (RCN, 2004). Initially, controlled drugs were also excluded from PGDs; but in October 2003 the Home Office issued a circular (HOC 49/2003: Home Office 2003) that contained amendments to the Misuse of Drugs Act 1971 and thus allows the supply and administration of certain controlled drugs, for example diamorphine for cardiac pain, which can be administered by Emergency Nurses and those who work in a Coronary Care Unit (CCU).

One of the most important aspects of the use of medicines within a PGD relating to a specific condition or situation is the inclusion of antimicrobials, and involving a local microbiologist for guidance and advice is strongly recommended. This guidance will ensure that the inclusion of an antimicrobial can be justified and that there will be minimal or no risk to any strategies already in place to combat antibiotic resistance (MeReC 2004).

Other factors to consider in the description of treatment are the quantity, pharmaceutical strength and form, route of administration and frequency and range of dosages to be used. The dosage documented should be appropriate for the clinical condition, and the clinical criteria for selected doses should be specified. First-line treatments for first episodes should be included as well as any additional treatments required. The individual using the PGD should record in the patient notes the name, dose, route of administration and duration of treatment of medicine used, as well as signing and printing name and designation.

Advice must be given verbally and/or in written form before and after treatment, and must include the giving of a Patient Information Leaflet – this is in line with the EC Labelling and Leaflet Directive 92/27, which applies to all supplies of medicines (RPSGB 2004).

- *Management and monitoring of PGDs* – It is important to document within the PGD all those who have been involved in the drawing up and approval process of the PGD. Demonstration of documentation to support an audit trail is also a pre-requisite, which allows information gathered regarding the correct implementation and use of the PGD to be easily accessible. Another important amendment to the original criteria is the arrangement for the security and storage of medicine, including the ability 'to reconcile incoming stock and outgoings on a patient by patient basis' (NHS Executive, 2000: HSC 2000/026, no. 9). The authors use a reconciliation book for each medicine given out to a patient – this involves documentation of patient details, how much medicine was given, the date the medicine was given and the total outstanding medicine left against the original stock number – in principle the documentation is very similar to a Controlled Drug register.

The expiry date of the PGD must be agreed and included in this section of the PGD – current guidance suggests that a PGD should be reviewed every two years, or more frequently in cases involving a particular use of some medicines (NHS Executive, 2000: HSC 2000/026). The PGD must be reviewed and resubmitted for approval to use before its expiry date, otherwise it becomes no longer valid and medicines cannot be administered or supplied under an expired PGD. The NPC (2004) states that all documentation for PGDs should be kept for eight years for adults, and, in the case of children, either until the child has reached its twenty-fifth birthday or until eight years after the child has died.

THE DEVELOPMENT OF PGDS

As has already been mentioned, a multidisciplinary team approach is important in the process of the creation of a PGD, and should include the healthcare professional(s) who will be administering and supplying medication, as well as a senior doctor and a senior pharmacist. If the PGD requires the administration and/or supply of an antimicrobial then the expertise of a microbiologist or public health specialist must be sought. Before use, the PGD must be authorised by the organisation in which the PGD will be used, for example the relevant NHS Trust or PCT, and all signatures should be documented – those who produced the PGD and those authorising its use, which may include a local Drugs Committee and a named Clinical Governance Lead.

IMPLEMENTATION OF PGDS

The named healthcare professional(s) who will be using the PGD must be able to demonstrate competency in the safe supply and/or administration of medicines – this must include documented evidence of skills and enhancement of professional knowledge undertaken with relevance to the clinical condition(s) that applies within the PGD. All healthcare professionals must act accordingly within their appropriate Code of Professional Conduct and have a complete understanding that they are professionally and personally accountable for their practice when using PGDs.

The Nursing and Midwifery Council (NMC) state: '*as a registered nurse, midwife or specialist community public health nurse, you are accountable for your actions and omissions. In administering any medication . . . you must exercise your professional judgement and apply your knowledge and skill in the given situation*' (NMC 2004a p. 4).

COMPETENCY

Healthcare professionals who use PGDs must be able to demonstrate a level of competency in achieving safe clinical practice, and this may be demonstrated within an assessment framework. The devised framework for assessment should incorporate set goals for the individual to achieve as well as any professional, personal and ethical considerations regarding their practice. Flint and Scott (2003) have developed their own competency framework for assessing an individual using a PGD, and the framework incorporates practical as well as theoretical issues – these include inclusion and exclusion criteria, information-giving, and, most importantly, the process by which individuals can identify their own learning needs.

Another competency framework tool relating to PGDs has been published by the National Prescribing Centre (NPC, 2004). It is a comprehensive document, and can be adapted to suit local and national needs and guidelines, as well as providing a valuable tool to aid the individual's reflection of practice of using PGDs. Areas discussed within the framework include:

- Clinical and pharmaceutical knowledge
- Establishing options
- Communicating with patients
- Safe PGD use
- Professional standards
- Practice development
- Information in context
- The NHS in context
- The Team and Individual in context

INDEPENDENT PRESCRIBING

In 1986 the Cumberlege Report (DHSS 1986) recommended that there should be a limited list of items that could be prescribed by nurses. These recommendations were reviewed by the Department of Health in the first Crown Report (DH, 1989). In 1998 nurse prescribing was introduced in England for district nurses and health visitors as a result of changes in legislation between 1992 and 1994. This enabled them to prescribe from a limited formulary of dressings and appliances and some medicines. Following the Review of the Prescribing, Supply and Administration of Medicines (the second Crown Report, DH 1999) the Department of Health introduced a more comprehensive formulary for independent nurse prescribing that broadened the scope for independent and supplementary prescribing and also allowed all first-level registered nurses to undertake training to become prescribers. This formulary is known as The Nurse Prescribers' Extended Formulary (NPEF; www.bnf.org) and lists the specific medical conditions that nurses can prescribe for, and the medicines that they can prescribe.

Recent research, carried out by the University of Southampton (DH, 2005a), found that independent nurse prescribing was viewed positively by patients, doctors and nurses themselves, with patients citing accessibility as a major advantage when obtaining their medicine from a nurse rather than a doctor. The research evaluated the first two years of extended formulary nurse prescribing and used a national survey, observation of prescribing nurses and the views of stakeholders in its assessment. Nurse prescribing is a registerable training, and nurses may not prescribe without being registered with the Nursing and Midwifery Council (NMC).

John Reid, as health secretary in 2003, stated that 'by opening the prescription pad to nurses we have given them a powerful and symbolic tool. One that makes choice a reality for patients' (Lanyon, 2004).

Adams (2004) considers the ability to prescribe medications as creating an inequality between the prescriber and the patient. He considers this a power inequality, and goes on to analyse the ethical dimensions of how this power is used by the prescriber. Prescribing treatment is a step further for nursing, as it allows nurses greater independence, enabling them to practise their craft with greater autonomy and freedom; but as with all freedom, this comes with a responsibility to use that freedom and autonomy in a way that benefits patients and society.

The Department of Health had a vision of 10,000 nurse prescribers by the end of 2004 . . . by November 2004, there were 5,000 (Ring 2004).

TRAINING

Nurse prescribing requires commitment and resources from employers as well as support and leadership for nurse prescribers. It is essential that all nurses who wish to undertake training to become independent or supplementary prescribers must be registered with the Nursing and Midwifery Council (NMC).

The NMC has now determined a new standard in respect of Independent Prescribing (for the Extended Formulary) and Supplementary Prescribing, and will only validate new recordable courses against this standard. To enable modification of existing Extended Formulary nurse prescribing courses, additional training and preparation has been incorporated to form the new NMC standard for Independent and Supplementary Prescribing at academic level 3.

The Department of Health believes that preparation for supplementary prescribing will take between one and two additional days, together with the course on Extended Formulary nurse prescribing. It was therefore decided that the length of a combined course covering both the Nurse Prescribers' Extended Formulary and Supplementary Prescribing should be at least 26 days, plus learning in practice. Of the 26 days' taught element, a substantial proportion should be face-to-face contact time. However, other ways of learning, such as open- and distance-learning formats, are also being considered for future development.

The NMC has requirements for validation of extended independent nurse prescribing and supplementary prescribing courses. The standard of the programme should be at a level no less than first degree, and a variety of assessment strategies should be used that should focus upon the principles and practice of prescribing, professional accountability and responsibility of the practitioners on the council's register.

The principal areas, knowledge and competencies are in the following table taken from the NMC (NMC 2004b):

Table 22

Principal areas	Knowledge	Competence
Principles	Legislation that underpins prescribing	• Works within the legislative framework relevant to the area of practice and locality. • Understands the principles behind supplementary prescribing and how they are applied to practice. • Able to use adverse reaction reporting mechanisms.
	Team working principles and practice	• Aware of the impact of prescribing in the wider delivery of care. • Able to work and communicate as part of a multidisciplinary prescribing workforce. • Reviews diagnosis and generates treatment options within the clinical treatment management plan.
	Philosophy and psychology of prescribing	• Understands the complexity of the external demands and influences on prescribing.

Table 22 *Continued*

Principal areas	Knowledge	Competence
Practice	Up-to-date clinical and pharmaceutical knowledge	• Makes an accurate assessment and diagnosis and generates treatment options. • Relevant to own area of expertise.
	Principles of drug dosage, side-effects, reactions and interactions	• Able to prescribe safely, appropriately and cost-effectively. • Understands how medicines are licensed.
	Communication, consent and concordance	• Able to work with patients and clients as partners in treatment. • Proactively develops dynamic clinical management plans. • Able to assess when to prescribe and when to make appropriate referral. • Able to refer back to medical practitioner when appropriate.
	Relationship of public health to prescribing	• Aware of policies that have an impact on public health and influence prescribing practice. • Able to articulate the boundaries of prescribing practice in relation to the duty of care to patients and society.
Accountability	The code of professional conduct The lines of accountability at all levels for prescribing	• Able to apply the principles of accountability to prescribing practice. • Able to account for the costs and effects of prescribing practice. • Regularly reviews evidence behind therapeutic strategies.
	Drug abuse and the potential for misuse	• Able to assess risk to the public of inappropriate use of prescribed substances.
	Requirements of record-keeping	• Understands where and how to access and use patient/client record. • Able to write and maintain coherent records of prescribing practice.
	Lines of communication	• Able to communicate effectively with patients, clients and professional colleagues.
Responsibility	Leadership skills	• Able to advise and guide peers in the practice of prescribing.
	Roles of other prescribers	• Able to articulate and understand the roles of other key stakeholders in prescribing practice.

Table 22 *Continued*

Principal areas	Knowledge	Competence
	Relationship of prescribers to pharmacists	• Understands the requirements of pharmacists in the prescribing and supply process.
	Clinical governance requirements in prescribing practice	• Links prescribing practice with evidence base, employer requirements and local formularies.
	Audit trails to inform prescribing practice	• Demonstrates ability to audit practice, undertake reflective practice and identify continuing professional development needs.

SUPERVISED LEARNING IN PRACTICE

There is a requirement from the Department of Health that a period of supervised practice and learning should form part of the preparation to become a nurse prescriber. The Department of Health states that: '*For the nurse/midwife, supervised learning will cover a total of 12 days spread over a 3 month period*' (DH, 2004).

There are also a number of requirements of the supervisor:

(i) The supervisor will be a doctor who has had three years recent experience for a group of patients in a relevant clinical field

(ii) (a) The doctor will be a General Practitioner with either vocational training or certification from the Joint Committee for Post Graduate Training in General Practice

Or

(b) A specialist registrar, clinical assistant or consultant within a NHS Trust or other NHS employer

(iii) The supervisor must have the support of the employing organisation or GP practice to act as the designated medical practitioner who will provide supervision, support and opportunities to develop competence in prescribing practice

(iv) Has some experience or training in teaching or supervising in practice.

MAINTAINING COMPETENCY

In 2001 the National Prescribing Centre published a document that outlined a framework of competencies a nurse prescriber should have (NPC 2001). The framework was intended to help individual nurse prescribers and their managers identify gaps in knowledge and skills and training needs to inform education and training for nurse prescribers and to support professionals locally by providing a framework to help the recruitment and selection procedure and to inform appraisal systems.

The framework is made up of various components:

- The main areas of competency
    1. The consultation
    2. Prescribing effectively
    3. Prescribing in context

Each of these areas has three different competencies, and each competency has:
1. An overarching statement, which gives an overall picture of what the competency is about
2. A number of statements, known as behavioural indicators, which represent the specific behaviours you would expect to see if the competency is applied effectively

The framework is summarised below:

Table 23

The Consultation		
Clinical and pharmaceutical knowledge	Establishing options	Communication with patients
Has up-to-date clinical and pharmaceutical knowledge relevant to own area of practice.	Makes a diagnosis and generates treatment options for the patient. Always follows up treatment.	Establishes a relationship based on trust and mutual respect. Sees patients as partners in the consultation. Applies the principles of concordance.
Prescribing effectively		
Prescribing safely	Prescribing professionally	Improving prescribing practice
Is aware of own limitations. Does not compromise patient safety.	Works within professional and organizational standards. Takes responsibility for prescribing decisions.	Actively participates in the review and development of prescribing practice.

Table 23 *Continued*		
Prescribing in context		
Information in context	The NHS in context	The team and individual context
Knows how to access relevant information. Can critically appraise and apply information in practice.	Understands, and works with local and national policies that impact on prescribing practice.	Works in partnership with colleagues to benefit patients. Is self-aware and confident in own ability as a prescriber.

THE FUTURE

Non-medical prescribing is an area that is changing rapidly. At the time of writing, the Department of Health was undertaking a consultation exercise regarding options for expanding independent nurse prescribing (DH, 2005b). The Evaluation of Extended Formulary Independent Nurse Prescribing carried out by the University of Southampton (DH, 2005a) found that the vast majority of nurses considered the limited formulary placed unhelpful limitations on their practice, and on 10 November 2005 the health secretary announced the results of this consultation.

The press statement stated:

> *From spring 2006, qualified Extended Formulary nurse prescribers and pharmacist independent prescribers will be able to prescribe any licensed medicine for any medical condition – with the exception of controlled drugs* (DH, 2005c).

REFERENCES

Adams J (2004) *Prescribing: The Ethical Dimension.* Published 14/07/04, available at: www.nurse-prescriber.co.uk

British National Formulary, available at: www.bnf.org

DH (Department of Health) (1989) *Report of the Advisory Group on Nurse Prescribing (Crown Report).* DH, London

DH (Department of Health) (1998) *A Report on the Supply and Administration of Medicines under Group Protocol (Crown Report, Part 1).* DH, London

DH (Department of Health) (1999) *Review of Prescribing, Supply and Administration of Medicines (Crown II) Final Report.* DH, London

DH (Department of Health) (2004) *Supervised Learning in Practice*, available at: www.dh.gov.uk

DH (Department of Health) (2005a) *An Evaluation of the Extended Formulary Independent Nurse Prescribing.* University of Southampton, DH, London

DH (Department of Health) (2005b) *Consultation on Options for the Future of Independent Prescribing by Extended Formulary Nurse Prescribers,* available at: www.dh.gov.uk

DH (Department of Health) (2005c) *Press release on the results of the consultation on Extended Formulary Independent Nurse Prescribing.* Available at: www.dh.gov.uk

DHSS (Department of Health and Social Security) (1986) *Neighbourhood Nursing: A Focus for Care. Report of the Community and Nursing Review (the Cumberlege Report).* HMSO, London

Flint H, Scott L (2003) Patient Group Directions: training practitioners for competency *Nursing Times* 99 (22) (June) 30–2

Gilmour C, Bickford J, Bruton J, Sullivan A, Davidson I (2005) *Patient Group Direction for Nurse Practitioner Supply of Drug Treatment for Genital Candidiasis in the Genitourinary Medicine Clinics of the HIV/GU Directorate (unpublished).* London: Chelsea and Westminster HC Trust

Home Office (2003) *An Amendment to the Misuse of Drugs Relations 2001 – To permit the Prescribing of controlled drugs by nurses in restricted circumstances, and the Supply of controlled drugs in accordance with a Patient Group Direction HOC 49/2003.* London: Home Office. Available from: <http://www.circulars.homeoffice. gov.uk> (accessed 10 October 2005)

Lanyon M (2004) *Nurse Prescribing: Current Status and Future Developments. Nursing Times* 100 (17, April)

McHale J (2003) A review of the legal framework for accountable nurse prescribing. *Nurse Prescribing* 1 (3) (August) 107–12

MeReC (2004) Supplementary Prescribing and Patient Group Directions. *MeReC Briefing Issue no. 23* (National Prescribing Centre March 1–8). Available from: <http://www.npc.co.uk/MeReC_Briefings/2003/briefing_no_23.pdf> (accessed 10 October 2005)

MHRA (2000) *Sale, supply and administration of medicines by health professionals under patient group directions (MLX 260).* MHRA, London

MHRA (2005) *Availability, prescribing, selling and supplying of medicines.* MHRA, London. Available from: <http://mhra.gov.uk/home/> (accessed 10 October 2005)

NHS Executive (1998) *Review of Prescribing, Supply and Administration of Medicines* HSC 1998/051. Department of Health, London

NHS Executive (2000) *Patient Group Directions (England Only) HSC 2000/026.* Department of Health, London

NMC (Nursing and Midwifery Council) (2004a) *Guidelines for the administration of medicines.* Nursing and Midwifery Council, London

NMC (Nursing and Midwifery Council) (2004b) *The council's requirements for 'Extended nurse prescribing and supplementary prescribing'* (available at www.dh.gov.uk)

NPC (National Prescribing Centre) (2001) *Maintaining Competency in Prescribing.* National Prescribing Centre, NHS, London

NPC (National Prescribing Centre) (2004) *Patient Group Directions – A practical guide and framework of competencies for all professionals using patient group directions* (National Prescribing Centre). Available from: <http://www.npc.nhs.uk/publications/pgd/pdg.htm> (accessed 10 October 2005)

RCN (Royal College of Nursing) (2004) *Patient Group Directions – Guidance and Information for Nurses* RCN, London

Ring M (2004) *Implementing nurse prescribing – the challenges.* Published 10/11/2004 (available at www.nurse-prescriber.co.uk)

RPSGB (Royal Pharmaceutical Society of Great Britain) (2004) *Fitness to Practice and Legal Affairs Directorate Fact Sheet Ten: Patient Group Directions.* RPSGB, London. Available from: <http://www.rpsgb.org/pdfs/factsheet10.pdf> (accessed 10 October 2005)

Statutory Instrument (2000) *The Prescription Only Medicines (Human Use) Amendment Order 2000.* Statutory Instrument No. 1917. HMSO, London

Statutory Instrument (2000) *The Medicines (Sale or Supply) (Miscellaneous Provisions) Amendment (no. 2) Regulations 2000.* Statutory Instrument No. 1918. HMSO, London

Statutory Instrument (2000) *The Medicines (Pharmacy and General Sale Exemption) Amendment Order 2000.* Statutory Instrument No. 1919. HMSO, London

Index

Page numbers in italic refer to tables or figures.

Advanced Clinical Skills for GU Nurses. Edited by Matthew Grundy-Bowers and Jonathan Davies
© 2007 John Wiley & Sons Ltd